Heal
with Oil

By Rebecca Park Totilo

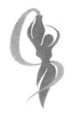

Heal with Oil

Printed in the United States of America.

Published by Rebecca at the Well Foundation, PO Box 60044, St. Petersburg, Florida 33784.

Disclaimer Notice: The information contained in this book is intended for educational purposes only and is not meant to substitute for medical care or prescribe treatment for any specific health condition. Please see a qualified health care provider for medical treatment. We assume no responsibility or liability for any person or group for any loss, damage or injury resulting from the use or misuse of any information in this book. No express or implied guarantee is given regarding the effects of using any of the products described herein.

ISBN 978-0974911540

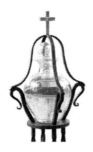

Contents

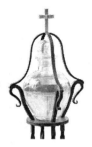

Introduction

Many of the most highly praised fragrances and essential oils are presented in Holy Scripture. These include Spikenard, Galbanum, Frankincense, Myrrh, Cypress, Cedarwood, Aloes, Rose of Sharon, Cassia, Cinnamon, Hyssop, Onycha, Myrtle and many others.

Since ancient times, spices and oils have been an integral part of the Hebraic culture. People of the Holy Land understood the use of essential oils in maintaining wellness and physical healing, as well as the oils' ability to enhance their spiritual state in worship, prayer and confession, and for cleansing and purification from sin. During biblical times, essential oils were inhaled, applied to the body, and taken internally in which the benefits extended to every aspect of their being.

Most Jewish households employed essential oils for medicinal and household purposes. One example in scripture is the parable Yeshua (Jesus) told of the Good Samaritan, who was carrying oil and wine and helped the injured man that had been robbed and left for dead.

Essential oils can be emotionally, spiritually, mentally, and physically healing and transform diseased tissue into thriving, healthy cells. Unfortunately, people today have become dependent and rely heavily on medicine. In many cases, it helps, but for most their faith has been placed in doctors instead of the Creator. In an article entitled "Death by Medicine," published by Nutrition Institute of America, four doctors stated that almost 800,000 deaths occur each year due to drug interaction.

The scriptures show that God gave natural herbs, including their extracts, for medicines. Ezekiel 47:12 reads:

> *And by the river upon the bank thereof, on this side and on that side, shall grow all trees for meat, whose leaf shall not fade, neither shall the fruit thereof be consumed: it shall bring forth new fruit according to his months, because their waters they issued out of the sanctuary: and the fruit thereof shall be for meat, and the leaf thereof for medicine.*

Moreover, in Revelation 22:2, it says:

> *In the midst of the street of it, and on either side of the river, was there the tree of life, which bare twelve manner of fruits, and yielded her fruit every month: and the leaves of the tree were for the healing of the nations.*

Essential oils of the Bible come from plant essences and are considered the life-blood of the plant. The two types of oils plants make are essential and fatty. Most seeds contain both types of oils. Essential oils circulate within a plant to carry out its function as a living creation while the fatty oils remain in the seed where they serve as food for the young plant, as God intended. Fragrant essential oils help plants communicate to the rest of the animal kingdom and humanity. Plants use their odors to attract insects and animals to pollinate, with fragrances disappearing within 30 minutes of being pollinated.

While fatty vegetable oil from the seed serves as nourishment for the small plant, it cannot enter the bloodstream nor cross the blood-brain barrier in humans. The molecules of fatty oils are too large to evaporate and circulate through the tissues of the body. Their uses in aromatherapy are for providing a neutral lipid base in which essential oils can be blended and/or diluted for massage use when an essential oil is too strong.

Essentials oils were God's original medicine, created on the third day. When God created these plants, His word went forth in power creating life and continues to create life in the life-blood of the plant, which is the oil. Genesis 1:12-13 says:

> *And the earth brought forth grass, and herb yielding seed after his kind and the tree yielding fruit, whose seed was in itself, after his kind: and God saw that it was good. And the evening and the morning were the third day.*

In this book, we will cover the various aspects of essential oils used in ancient times, their history, spiritual significance, and their healing properties.

SPICE CHEST: A HOLY PRIESTHOOD

God gave Moses instructions for which specific fragrances to use for making the holy anointing oil in Exodus 30:22-31:

> Moreover, the LORD spake unto Moses saying, Take thou also unto thee principal spices, of pure Myrrh five hundred shekels, and of sweet Cinnamon half so much, even two hundred and fifty shekels, and of sweet calamus two hundred and fifty shekels, and of Cassia five hundred shekels, after the shekel of the sanctuary, and of oil Olive an hin: and thou shalt make it an oil of holy ointment, an ointment compound after the art of the apothecary: it shall be an holy anointing oil. And thou shalt anoint the tabernacle of the congregation therewith, and the ark of the testimony, and the table and all his vessels, and the candlestick and his vessels, and the altar of incense, and the altar of burnt offering with all his vessels, and the laver and his foot. And thou shalt sanctify them, that they may be most holy: whatsoever toucheth them shall be holy. And thou shalt anoint

Aaron and his sons, and consecrate them, that they may minister unto me in the priest's office. And thou shalt speak unto the children of Israel, saying, This shall be an holy anointing oil unto me throughout your generations.

During the Mosaic period, certain oils were designated by God as the holy anointing oil to sanctify the Hebraic genealogy known as the Cohanim priests. This ritual anointing performed on these priests distinguished them not only for Temple service, but also, according to Rabbi Aryeh Kaplan, registered and changed the DNA of their cells, which has continued throughout all generations.

According to an article entitled "Lost Tribes of Israel," Nova Online reported on the existence of a distinctive Y chromosome in the DNA of Aaron's descendants:

"Genetic studies among Cohanim from all over the world reveal the truth behind this oral tradition. About 50 percent of Cohanim in both Sephardic and Ashkenazic populations have an unusual set of genetic markers on their Y chromosome. What is equally striking is that this genetic signature of the Cohanim is rarely found outside the Jewish populations."

They also stated that rabbis at the Western Wall in Jerusalem took swab tests of Jewish males desiring to know if they were a part of the tribe of Levi in preparation for the third temple.

THE ANCIENT ART OF EXTRACTING OILS

In ancient times, essential oils and other aromatics were used for religious rituals, as well as for the treatment of illness and other physical and spiritual needs. According to the *Essential Oils Desk Reference* compiled by Essence Science Publishing, "Records dating back to 4500 B.C. describe the use of balsamic substances with aromatic properties for religious rituals and medical applications. The translation of ancient papyrus found in the Temple of Edfu, located on the west bank of the Nile, reveals medicinal formulas and perfume recipes used by the alchemist and high priest in blending aromatic substances for rituals performed in the temples and pyramids."

As well, hieroglyphics on the walls of Egyptian temples depict the blending of oils and describe hundreds of oil recipes. These writings tell of scented barks, resins of spices, and aromatic vinegar, wines and beers that were used in rituals, temples, embalming and medicine. Thus, the Egyptians were credited as the first to discover the potential of fragrance and were considered masters in using essential oils and other aromatics in the embalming process. They created various aromatic blends for personal use, placing them in alabaster jars – a vessel specially carved and shaped for holding fragrant oils. In fact, when King Tut's tomb was opened in 1922, 350 liters of oils were discovered in alabaster jars. Amazingly, because of the solidification of plant waxes sealing the opening of the jars, the liquefied oil was in perfect condition.

In the upper region of Egypt was a sect of Jews, called Essenes, who were known for their healing arts and use of essential oils. Both Philo and Josephus' writings indicated that at the period in which John the Baptist and Jesus were born, the Essenes were scattered over Palestine, numbering about four thousand souls. The term *Essenes*, or *Therapeuts* (used interchangeably), refers primarily to the art of healing which these devotees professed, as it was believed in those days that sanctity was closely allied to the exercise of this power and that no cure of any sort could be imputed simply to natural ets.org)

According to Miriam Stead, author of *Egyptian Life*, the process of steam distillation was not known for the extraction of essences, but there were three techniques available for producing perfumes from flowers, fruits, and seeds. She writes of one method: "There was enfleurage, the saturation of layers of fat with perfume by steeping flowers in the fat and replacing them when their perfume was spent. In this way, the Egyptians were able to create creams and pomades."

THE ORIGINAL CONEHEADS

A popular form of pomade was the so-called cosmetic cone, which was worn on top of the head. Those frequently represented in banqueting scenes were worn by guests and servants alike. The cone was usually white with streaks of orange-brown running from its top. Its coloring represented the perfume with which the cone was impregnated. As the evening progressed, the cone would melt and the scented oil would run down over the wig and garment, creating a pleasing scent, but no doubt a sticky mess. Throughout the course of an evening, it became necessary to renew the scent on the cones. The tomb scenes show servants circulating among the guests replenishing the perfumed cream.

A favorite late-night comedy television show, *Saturday Night Live*, used to include a skit of a family with coneheads. While the writers of this routine thought they were original, cone-shaped heads were all the rage in ancient Egypt.

A second process for creating perfume was maceration, dipping flowers, herbs or fruits into fats or oils heated to a temperature of about 65 degrees Celsius. This technique is depicted in a number of tomb scenes. The flowers or fruits were pounded in mortars and then stirred into the oil, which was kept hot on a fire. The mixture was sieved and allowed to cool, so that it could be shaped into balls or cones, or if in liquid form, poured into vessels. An alternative process may have been to macerate the flowers in water, cover the vessel with a cloth impregnated with fat, and boil the contents of the container until all the perfumes had evaporated, fixing them in the fat which was then scraped off the cloth. This technique is still used by peoples living near the source of the Nile.

There was also the possibility of expressing the flowers or seeds. This process was borrowed from the manufacture of wine and oil. The material to be pressed was placed in a bag with a stick attached to each end. The rods were twisted by a group of workmen. This technique was not often used as most recipes specified either maceration or enfleurage.

HOW ESSENTIAL OILS ARE PRODUCED TODAY

Producing essential oil continues to take much work. It takes sixty thousand rose blossoms to produce one ounce of Rose oil, whereas lavender is easier to obtain and yields approximately seven pounds of oil from two hundred and twenty pounds of dried flowers. The Sandalwood tree must be thirty years old and over thirty feet tall before it can be cut down for distillation. Myrrh, Frankincense, and Benzoin oils are extracted from the gum resins of their respective trees, while citrus fruits such as Orange, Lemon and Lime are squeezed from the peel of their fruits. Cinnamon essential oil comes from the bark of the tree (and leaves as well), and Pine oil comes from the needles and twigs. Other flowers must be picked by hand early in the morning before the sun rises and heats them, evaporating the essential oil within their petals. Hence, production affects the variation in pricing of various essential oils on the market.

There is a variety of ways in which essential oils are extracted. The most common methods are steam distillation, solvent extraction, expression, enfleurage, and maceration.

Steam distillation involves using steam to pull essential oils from the plant by suspending the plant material over water in a sealed container, which is then brought to a boil. The steam containing the volatile essential oil is run through a cooler, and when it condenses the liquid is collected. The essential oil appears as a thin film on top of the liquid, as water and essential oils do not mix. The essential oil is then separated from the water by collecting it in a small vial, while the water collects in a large vat.

Solvent extraction involves using very little heat to preserve the oil, which would otherwise be destroyed or altered during steam distillation. The plant material is dissolved in a liquid solvent of heptane, hexane, or methylene chloride as a suitable perfume solvent, which absorbs the smell, color, and wax of the plant. After removing the plant material, the solvent is boiled off under a vacuum to help separate the essential oil from it. This can be achieved as the solvent evaporates quicker, leaving a substance called 'concrete.' The concrete is mixed in with alcohol to aid in filtering the waxes. The next process involves distilling the alcohol away, which leaves an 'absolute.' The word 'absolute' appears on the label of some bottled essential oils although they still contain 2-3 percent of the solvent; therefore, these oils are not considered pure essential oil.

Expression is used for citrus oils rather than distillation. Within citrus fruits such as Orange, Lemon, Lime and Grapefruit, the essential oil is located in little sacs just under the surface of the rind. The oils need to be squeezed out, or expressed, from the peels and seeds. This is achieved by letting the fruit roll over a conveyor covered in small needles that pierce the little oil pockets in the citrus rind. The oil runs out and is caught and filtered.

Enfleurage is an ancient method of extracting oils that is rarely used today because of its long, complicated and expensive process. Fragrant blooms were placed upon sheets of warm animal fat (or long layers of vegetable fat), which absorbed the essential oil. As flowers are exhausted, they are replaced with fresh blossoms. This process is repeated until the sheet of fat is saturated with fragrance and is separated with solvents, leaving only the essential oil.

Maceration is the process of macerating, but does not produce pure essential oils as they are mixed with carrier oils. Plant material is gathered and chopped, then added to either Sunflower or Olive oil. The mixture is stirred for a while and then placed in the sunlight for several days. This process brings out all of the soluble components in the plant material, including the essential oil, which is then carefully filtered. This process leaves a carrier oil infused with essential oil.

ESSENTIAL OILS AS GOD'S MEDICINE

The leaf thereof is for medicine. Ezekiel 47:12

Aromatherapy is a branch of alternative medicine that uses specific "aromas" from essential oils that have curative effects. The healing art of aromatherapy traces back to 4000-5000 B.C. when the Egyptians, Greeks, Hebrews, Romans and Persians burned herbs and flowers for medicinal purposes. Today, many are rediscovering those ancient healing practices as a path back to divine health.

Within each plant's oil is the complex makeup of 200-800 chemical constituents. Because of the variability and unpredictability of these constituents, pathogenic microorganisms such as bacteria and viruses are unable to build up a resistance to them in their efforts of mutation against essential oils. Synthetic drugs that are made by isolating one or two constituents are no match for bacteria or a virus, which can quickly adapt and mutate, rendering the drugs useless. There are simply too many constituents within an essential oil for a virus to adapt to. In fact, many essential oils prove to be more effective than antibiotics and possess the intelligence to leave the beneficial bacteria untouched. Chemist and Aromatherapy Practitioner Dr. Kurt Schnaubelt states essential oils have a 95% success potential against infections.

In an online article entitled "Essential Oils: For Cold Care and a Strong Immune System," Misty Rae Cech, ND author writes, "Because of their chemical composition, essential oils can be easily absorbed into the human body, passing through cell membranes, then into the bloodstream due to their 'lipophilic' nature (a structure in alignment with the lipid components of the body's cell walls). Essential oils can protect us from microbes in many different ways, from keeping the space around us naturally microbe-free to readying our immune system for defense, to destroying the microbes once they've entered our bodies."

Simply by diffusing essential oils into the atmosphere, the oils eliminate microbes in the air, thus reducing the concentration of live pathogens you may inhale or touch at any time lessening the load on your immune system. Second, most essential oils, especially the strong antimicrobial ones, have an uplifting effect on the psyche and a sharpening impact on the mind. Finally, essential oils can fortify your immune system to prevent you from catching an illness in the first place –some studies that have shown mammalian cells having increased resistance to microbial invaders after exposure to essential oils.

While essential oils' powerful weapon of antimicrobial compounds equips us against viral pathogens that attempt to invade the body, most agree essential oils are not "wonder drugs." Conventional medicine has its place, and should certainly be employed when it will provide the best results. Alternative medicine, such as aromatherapy, offers a suitable resolution in relation to its therapeutic value and can be effective if used sensibly and with sound judgment.

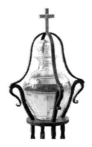

History of ESSENTIAL OILS

Historical records show that people's use of scents, aromas, fragrances, and essential oils have been in almost every culture for millennia and are considered man's first medicine. Essential oils and other forms of aromatics have been used in religious ceremonies, for treating various illnesses and for spiritual and emotional needs.

Ancient manuscripts record the use of medicinal herbs dating back to 2800 B.C., documenting the use of plants with aromatic qualities for healing by the Chinese and the Egyptians. The Ebers papyrus from the 18th dynasty listed herbal formulas for problems such as eye inflammation, which called for Myrrh, Cypress, and Frankincense. Other recipes recorded included a blend for deodorant using aromatics and treatments for depression and nervous disorders. The Egyptian priests used aromatics such as Cedarwood, Sandalwood, and Aloes in their embalming practices and for mummification.

While the Babylonians may have been the first to extravagantly perfume their mortar with which they built their temples, townships commissioned by the Pharaoh Akhenaton and Queen Nefertiti built large squares designated for the burning of herbs to keep the air fragrant and germ-free. Cleopatra, the Queen of Egypt, drenched the sails of her ships with the most exotic aromatic essential oils so that their essences would herald her arrival along the banks of the Nile. The Greeks quickly learned from the Egyptians and visited the Nile Valley, which later became known as the Cradle of Medicine, in 500 B.C.

The Greeks attributed sweet aromas to their gods with the burning of incense. Perfumery at this time was closely linked to religion and each god was allotted a fragrance. Statues were anointed with secret formulas made by their priests, and fragrant herbs and oils were used for anointing at times of prayer and for healing.

During biblical times, the Hebrews scattered fresh leaves and twigs of fresh mint and other herbs along the dirt floors of homes and synagogues so that as they walked on them, the aromatic essential oils would be released into the air. This practice was also common in the temple, where they sacrificed animals, allowing the scent to act as a disinfectant.

When the use of essential oils spread to Greece, they were not only used in religious ceremonies, but also for personal purposes, as well. Hippocrates, the father of medicine, was known for practicing an "ancient form" of aromatherapy. He recommended a daily bath regimen using essential oils for wellbeing. In Athens, he combated the bubonic plague by fumigating the whole city with fragrant essences from plants. Another Greek physician, Megallus, formulated an aromatic remedy called Megalleon made from Cinnamon, Myrrh, and charred Frankincense resins soaked in Balanos oil, which gained notoriety for its curative benefits as an anti-inflammatory and with healing wounds.

Because of the excessive use of aromatic oils, the demand for the raw materials necessary to produce both fragrances and remedies led to the discovery of new and more efficient ways for extraction. Such techniques as pressing, decoction, pulverization and maceration were developed and mastered by both the Assyrians and the Egyptians. They even made attempts to produce essential oils by distillation. Avicenna, a Persian in the 10th century, refined the process of distillation by inventing a machine with a coiled cooling pipe that allowed for more efficient cooling. Because of this, the focus eventually shifted towards more emphasis on true essential oils and their uses. Oil of Cedarwood distilled with such machines was used along with Myrrh, Cinnamon, Clove Bud and Nutmeg oils to embalm the dead. Also, they adopted the essential oils they distilled into medicine, cosmetics, and fragrances.

In an effort to outdo the Greeks, the Romans began to use essential oils more lavishly in their practices of therapeutic massage and personal hygiene. They used aromatics in steam baths to both rejuvenate their bodies and ward off disease. Dioscorides, a Roman, wrote a treatise on the uses of 500 different plant substances called "De Materia Medica." Many historical manuscripts ascribe to how herbs were brought from all over the world and distilled into essential oils. It was from this treatise the Roman herbalist Galen significantly influenced and wrote a medical reference that remained a standard for over 1,500 years. Later, Theophrastus wrote on odors and their influence on the mind and emotions.

Paracelsus, a doctor of the 15th century, coined the term "essence." His emphasis was the use of essential oils for medicine. He believed alchemy's role was in developing drugs and extracts from healing plants. During this time, many different essential oils were being produced. Among them were Juniper Berry, Rosemary, Rose, and Sage. Frequent visits to the local apothecary were made to buy essential oils for uses such as homeopathy, folk remedies, and healing rituals, as oils became a widely accepted part of health and medicine. Hence, the emergence of new essential oils flourished.

After the Roman Empire fell, the use of aromatics for personal consumption declined. It was not until the Middle Ages essential oils once again emerged, this time in the churches of Europe for religious ceremonies and to mask the reeking odor caused by disease, which abounded at that time. Essential oil extracts during the Dark Ages were valued for their antibacterial and antiviral properties. In the streets of Europe, garlands of fresh, aromatic herbs were worn while pine-scented candles and Frankincense were burned to conceal the stench of death and purify the air. Physicians wore heavy cloaks and large hats with a beak-like mask attached. Fragrant herbs were placed inside the beak, which purified the air they breathed. Also, they carried a large open-ended cane filled with herbs that they waved in front of them as they walked for extra protection. No doubt, they believed these essences protected them from the deadly pestilence.

With the advent of chemistry and chemical synthesis, natural forms of medicine became less popular until the beginning of the 20th century. The valuable curative properties of essential oils were not rediscovered until 1937 by a French chemist, Rene-Maurice Gattefosse. During a laboratory experiment, Gattefosse had an accident in which he suffered severe burns. He quickly immersed his hand into a nearby vat of pure Lavender essential oil that quickly healed his wounds. Gattefosse went on to extensively research essential oils and discovered their ability to penetrate the skin and enter into the body's internal organs and nervous system. He also classified the various effects of essential oils on the digestive system, the metabolism, the nervous system and the endocrine glands.

Another pioneer in the field of aromatherapy is Dr. Jean Valnet, a French scientist and army physician and surgeon, who used essential oils to successfully treat wounded soldiers during World War II when antibiotics ran out. His work established the development of the modern use of essential oils as a supplement to health care. Dr. Valnet's monumental work and theory of medicine founded on the natural therapeutic means continues to grow rapidly as health scientists and medical practitioners carry on research and validate the numerous benefits of essential oils for conventional medicine.

Today, the use of essential oils has become a significant part of the holistic approach to health and is ever-increasing across the planet. As many look for alternative ways to restore wellness, it is no surprise their search leads them back to the Holy Scriptures.

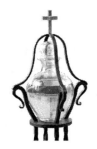

Oils of THE BIBLE

Journey back in time to the courts of the temple in Jerusalem, take a deep breath and inhale the aroma of the Holy Anointing Oil. Within the writ of Scripture, believers can find the recipe for health in the biblical fragrances – the root of man's search, which is key to unlocking the mysteries of healing.

Aromatic plants, herbs and essential oils have been used for aromatherapy, incense, perfume, culinary purposes and medicinal purposes for thousands of years by many cultures. The Bible mentions over 33 species of fragrant plants with over 1,035 references to essential oils and/or plants in the Old and New Testaments. God is obviously a lover of sweet, fragrant oils and perfumes. The Scriptures are filled with a plethora of fragrances in the context of anointing oils, perfume, spices, and incense. We find Frankincense referenced in sixteen verses in the Bible, Myrrh in seventeen verses, Spikenard mentioned in five verses, with many other references to Balsam Fir, Cinnamon, Cassia, Calamus, Henna, Stacte, Aloes, Onycha, Cedarwood, Hyssop, Pine, Pomegranates, Lilies, Rose of Sharon, and Saffron.

During biblical times, essential oils were inhaled, applied to the body as anointing oil, and taken internally in which the benefits extended to every aspect of their being physically, spiritually, emotionally, and mentally. David alluded to this in Psalm 51:7 when he wrote, *Purge me with Hyssop and I will be clean: Wash me, and I will be whiter than snow.* May your faith deepen and be enriched as you discover the hidden treasures and rich spiritual meaning of these exotic biblical fragrances!

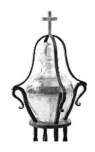

Acacia

Acacia plays a paralleled part in the Israelites history. In the Bible, its original name is Shittim. In the book of Exodus, Acacia is used to construct all of the structure features of the Tabernacle. Throughout this book's chapters, we find the Lord instructing Moses to use this valuable plant. It was used to make:

- The Ark and its poles
- The table of the showbread and its poles
- The brazen altar and its poles
- The poles for hanging the curtains

When we refer to the Semitic writings, Rashi in the Midrash (Rashi ibid 25:5) explains that this choice of plant, in particular, was no accident. On the contrary, its use was preordained many years before. Interestingly, one of the first things the Patriarch Jacob did when he entered Egypt was plant a Shittim for the Tabernacle 200 years later.

In Numbers 25:1 it says,

> *Israel settled in Shittim, and the people began to commit harlotry with the daughters of Moab.* They invited the people to the sacrifices of their gods, and the people ate and prostrated themselves to their gods.

The area and the fountain were called Shittim because of the abundance of trees surrounding it. However, if it was indeed a place of harlotry that watered Sodom (according to some translations) why would God want his house built there? Here the ancient Semitic sages teach a very similar philosophy to plant healers of today: The Lord makes the remedy before the illness, they say.

Another interpretation of this verse adds weight to these thoughts. The Gemara in Sanhedrin disputes the use of the word "settled" in this passage. When the original word *yashab* (and sometimes *vayeishev*) is used in the *Tanakh*, the Hebrew canon of the Bible, it always portrays difficulty and pain, or lack of growth and movement. This is an excellent depiction of the mental condition of the Israelites at that time. They had grown tired and weary of exile and had lost direction in their faith. It may be fair to say they had become stuck, and stagnation had set in; unfortunately, the opposite of progression is regression. Perhaps the sages were right. God made the antidote ready for when they arrived.

Indeed, Shittim seemed to have a very hallowed place in the Lord's heart. "God will return any Acacia (shittah) tree that gentiles took from Jerusalem," it says in the Babylonian Talmud, Rosh Hashanah 23:1. Even today, taking an Acacia tree from the desert is taboo. Aramaic tradition dictates anyone found doing so should suffer the penalty of having their arm cut off.

Acacia is an extremely resilient wood with its testament to the longevity of the Tabernacle. It stayed in situ until it was ensconced in the New Temple of Jerusalem built by Solomon over 400 years later. It was prized, too, it seems on a monetary basis.

When the Torah speaks of voluntary donation, Exodus 25:1-8 shows the high regard the Lord places on Acacia. No other wood was allowed, only the precious Acacia.

> *Tell the sons of Israel to raise a contribution for Me; from every man whose heart moves him, you shall raise My contribution. And this is the contribution which you are to raise from them: gold, silver and bronze, blue, purple and scarlet material, fine linen, goat hair, rams' skins dyed red, porpoise skins,* **Acacia wood,** *oil for lighting, spices for the anointing oil and for the fragrant incense, onyx stones and setting stones, for the ephod and for the breastpiece. And let*

*them construct a sanctuary for Me, that I
may dwell among them.*

But why Acacia? Why not some other prized wood? Apparently, for the most obvious reason, because it was there. In the arid dryness of the desert, few trees can grow. Acacia, however, thrives. Because of its tiny leaves, which conserve its water, these completely drop off during times when water is sparse.

Acadia is a very slow-growing crop. This means the wood grows to be extremely dense and hard. In the tree's heartwood, there are deposits that act as a preservative for the wood, repelling insects, but also hardly making the wood water. When it is polished, the heartwood becomes the most sumptuous reddish-brown color. The resin from the wood is the gum Arabic we know today. We see this also mentioned in the Old Testament called the medicine of the Acacia.

There seems to be much confusion as to exactly which Acacia species was the one of the Old Testament. Every commentator seems to have a different opinion. There is little wonder since there are over 1,300 species listed in the subspecies *Mimosoideae*, from the family *Fabaceae*. Most likely candidates seem to be *Acacia arabica* or *Acacia raddiana*.

BIBLICAL REFERENCES TO ACADIA (SHITTAH)

Exodus 25:5
Exodus 25:10
Exodus 25:13
Exodus 25:23
Exodus 25:28
Exodus 26:15
Exodus 26:26
Exodus 26:32
Exodus 26:37
Exodus 27:1
Exodus 27:6
Exodus 30:1
Exodus 30:5
Exodus 35:7
Exodus 35:24
Exodus 36:20
Exodus 36:31
Exodus 36:36
Exodus 37:1
Exodus 37:4
Exodus 37:10
Exodus 37:15
Exodus 37:25
Exodus 37:28
Exodus 38:1
Exodus 38:6
Deuteronomy 10:3
Isaiah 41:19

ACACIA SHITTAH'S HEALING PROPERTIES

The name Acacia originates from the Greek term *akis*, which means "sharp point," after its typically thorny nature. There are hundreds of varieties of Acacia within the *Fabaceae* family. The Acacia tree referred to in the Bible is thought to be *Acacia arabica* – also known as the Shittah tree or *Acacia nilotica* – which is native to Africa and the Holy Land.

All parts of this medium-sized tree are traditionally used for healing purposes in Ayurvedic medicine. The essential oil is produced from the flowers of the plant by solvent extraction. Its base note scent is deep, woody, balsamic and floral, which blends well with oils such as Lavender, Ylang Ylang, Citronella, Frankincense, Orange, and Cassia.

TRADITIONAL USES

Acacia has a strong biblical association as wood from the Shittah tree, which was used to build the Tabernacle and the Ark of the Covenant. The Acacia tree is also thought to be the "burning bush" described in the book of Exodus. The plant was traditionally used as an entheogen – a natural chemical used to induce an altered state of consciousness in religious rituals.

In ancient India, Acacia was used as a tonic for digestive complaints, inflammation, toothaches and skin problems. Throughout history, herbalists have used Acacia to cure a range of disorders from respiratory conditions such as coughs, colds, fevers, and pneumonia, to parasitic worms, skin diseases, diarrhea, intestinal pains and tooth decay. It was also used to treat urinary tract infections, leucorrhea, and gonorrhea. In South America, the bark and root of the Acacia tree are traditionally made into a psychoactive drink (Source: The Encyclopedia of Psychoactive Plants: Ethnopharmacology and its Applications, Ratsch, C.).

MEDICINAL USES

In modern aromatherapy, Acacia essential oil is recommended for treating problems relating to the skin or the nervous system. Its relaxing scent can help with nervous disorders, including stress, anxiety and depression. Its astringent properties can be beneficial in treating skin infections, sores, and inflammation.

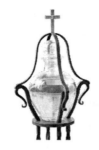

Aloes

There are two plants referred to as "Aloes" in the Bible. One is a rich, fragrant resin formed in the heartwood of the *Aquilaria* or Agarwood tree, in response to a natural parasite, fungal, or mold attack. This natural process happens when the logs are buried in the ground, and the outer part decays while the inner is saturated with this resin. The tree may also be deliberately wounded to make it susceptible to attack. Thus, the fungus and decomposition process can take over several hundred years to produce, making it one of the rarest and most expensive oils. Aloes is extremely scarce and costly. At the time of the writing of this book, a rotting log containing Agarwood was on sale on ebay.com for $65,000 USD.

The second reference to Aloes in the Bible is "lign Aloes" mentioned in Balaam's blessing for Israel. In Numbers 24:6 it says,

> As the valleys are they spread forth, as gardens by the river's side, as the trees of lign Aloes which the LORD hath planted, [and] as cedar trees beside the waters.

The Arabic word for Aloes in this verse means "little tents," derived from the triangular shape of the capsules from the lign Aloes trees, and its resin emits this fragrant spice. These "little tents" refer to a tent on the housetop – a place of intimacy or bridal tent. It was a common practice in the Middle East to build a small "honeymoon suite" on the rooftop of a house. 2 Samuel 16:22 tells how they "spread a tent on the top of the house" for Absalom. It is also mentioned in Song of Solomon 4:14. In Proverbs 7:17, this theme of Aloes referring to the place of intimacy says, *I have perfumed my bed with Myrrh, Aloes, and Cinnamon.*

In the New Testament, Aloes is only referenced once as a burial spice used in preparing Yeshua's body after his crucifixion. This rare fragrance employed is referenced in John 19:39:

> And there came also Nicodemus, which at the first came to Jesus by night, and brought a mixture of Myrrh and Aloes, about a hundred pound weight.

Intimacy again plays into this very tender story. Just before his death, Yeshua, like an Israeli bridegroom, comforted his disciples with these same words before he returned to his Father's house, spoken in the ancient Jewish rite in John 14:1-2:

> Let not your heart be troubled. In my Father's house are many mansions: if [it were] not [so], I would have told you. I go to prepare a place for you.

In ancient Israel, after the betrothal ceremony, the bridegroom left the bride's home and returned to his father's house to prepare for his wedding day. Before departing, he made a special promise to his bride: "I go and prepare a place for you, and when it is ready, I will return for you." During this time of separation, the groom built a bridal chamber or tent attached to his father's house, while the bride gathered her trousseau and made herself ready for his return.

BIBLICAL REFERENCES TO AGARWOOD (ALOES)

Number 24:6
Psalm 45:8
Proverbs 7:17
Song of Solomon 4:14
John 19:39

AGARWOOD'S HEALING PROPERTIES

Agarwood essential oil is derived from *Aquilaria* trees, which are native to India and Southeast Asia. When the heartwood becomes infected with a particular fungus, it causes the tree to produce an aromatic resin. Its rarity has led to Agarwood becoming one of the world's most expensive essential oils. Also known as Oud or Aloeswood, it belongs to the Thymelaeaceae botanical family.

The oil is steam distilled from the wood chips, producing a sweet, woody, base note fragrance that blends well with Sandalwood, Frankincense, Rose, Neroli, Jasmine,

Vetiver, and Geranium. Agarwood is not an oil that is commonly used in mainstream aromatherapy.

TRADITIONAL USES

Agarwood essential oil has been used as incense in religious ceremonies since ancient times. Known as the "wood of the Gods," it is still prescribed in Chinese medicine as a remedy for colds and digestive disorders. In traditional Ayurvedic medicine, Agarwood is considered to be a warming, stimulating oil that was traditionally used for gastrointestinal conditions, skin diseases, and bronchial asthma. Its use as an aphrodisiac is also noted throughout history. Burning Agarwood incense was commonly thought to clear the mind and prevent the spread of infection.

MEDICINAL USES

Agarwood has the ability to uplift the emotions and can be used to treat depression, stress, and anxiety. Its deep, woody fragrance can be very centering and useful for meditation. It can be helpful when treating urinary tract infections and menstrual disorders. Its antimicrobial properties can fight bronchitis and infectious skin conditions, such as acne. Agarwood is also known to support the nerves and circulation.

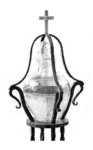

Almond

The almond has an indispensable part to play in both the symbolism in Hebrew teachings and actual recorded events. The almond tree was native to Syria and Palestine, and its Hebrew name *shaqedh* means "wakeful or hastening." It potentially received this name because of its urgency to flower in spring. White or very pale flowers spring from bare branches in February and sometimes as early as January, some years. However, it also has a second meaning of "to watch and wait" and this is used quite effectively in Scripture.

When the Lord speaks to Jeremiah, he asks him what he sees, and Jeremiah says,

> *And I said, I see a rod of an almond-tree (shaqedh). Then said Yahweh unto me, Thou hast well seen: for I will watch (shoqedh) over my word to perform it.*

What an omen! In this exquisite imagery of the bright white flowers lies a dark, threatening harbinger, because the Lord promises he is watching carefully as his people move further and further away from him, and it is only time before he raises his hand in judgment.

In Ecclesiastes 12:15, though, the use of the almond reference is an allegory of hastening toward old age before one's time and becoming fearful of life. The King James Version creates a grim picture:

> *Also, when they shall be afraid of that which is high, and fears shall be in the way, and the almond tree shall flourish, and the grasshopper shall be a burden, and desire shall fail: because man goeth to his long home, and the mourners go about the streets.*

Apparently, almonds held great monetary value during Old Testament times. It is suspected that almonds may not have grown in Egypt, only in Palestine, because in Genesis 43:11, Jacob tells his sons to take almonds with them. It is thought, then, that this delicacy held potential sway to secure Simeon and Benjamin's freedom. This almond "cultural" difference becomes paramount later in the story of the Exodus.

While Moses had grown up in an Egyptian court, Aaron instead was raised as a Canaanite. Aaron, Moses's older brother, a prophet of God, was mentioned several times throughout the Old Testament as wielding a staff; to the Hebrews, this would have been a sign of high authority. In early references, we read how he used the rod to shepherd sheep, but later it becomes an allegory for him leading his people. This staff had miraculous powers and is seen as powerful even without Aaron's command.

The first time we see this is when Moses commands Aaron to visit Pharaoh, who requires seeing a miracle. He tells him to cast down his staff in front of him. Aaron does this, and it turns into a serpent. The viziers and magicians of Pharaoh's court respond by casting down their own which also turn into snakes, but Aaron's serpent swallows them all, showing dominion over Egypt.

Later God commanded that each tribe should select a staff of a different wood and the one that blossomed would designate the tribe to become priests. Aaron planted his staff and when he entered the tent of meeting the next morning, not only had it flowered, but it had also born almonds, designating Aaron's tribe of Levi to be the chosen priesthood. Throughout their journey to the Promised Land, Aaron's staff helped the Israelites many times overcome the trials of the plagues.

This is later tested in the tabernacle, and again the staff performs the same way; it flowers and produces almonds, reaffirming the priesthood decision. This time, down one side grew bitter almonds and down the other side were sweet ones. For the Israelites, this meant that sweet almonds would flourish as long as they were faithful to their God, but the bitter almonds were a foreboding reminder of God's promise to Jeremiah. It is believed that the rod was later kept in the tabernacle in memorial of this.

SPICE CHEST: LIGHT OF THE WORLD

The tabernacle itself was a windowless tent, with all lighting coming from a candelabrum that God had commanded be built. The light from this beautiful menorah was to represent the Word of God, unnatural and otherworldly, and the lamp was fueled by a sacred blend of essential oils. It was made of solid gold and later depicted in Roman illustrations with the base as rectangular. We read in Exodus 25:32:

> *Six branches shall go out from its sides; three branches of the lampstand from its one side and three branches of the lampstand from its other side. Three cups shall be shaped like almond blossoms in the one branch, a bulb and a flower, and three cups shaped like almond blossoms in the other branch, a bulb and a flower – so for six branches*

going out from the lampstand; and in the lampstand four cups shaped like almond blossoms, its bulbs and its flowers.

Almonds are eaten at *Tu B'Shevat*, a holy day set aside as the Jewish New Year for plants. It falls in January or February on the Gregorian calendar, but in Israel, it marks the beginning of spring. Some scholars suggest that it may originally have been a folk festival to celebrate the emergence of spring.

BIBLICAL REFERENCES TO ALMOND

Genesis 30:37
Genesis 43:11
Exodus 25:33
Exodus 25:34
Exodus 37:19
Exodus 37:20
Numbers 17:2
Numbers 17:8
Jeremiah 1:11
Ecclesiastes 12:5

ALMOND'S HEALING PROPERTIES

Almond, which is not a nut but a drupe (a fruit with a nut-like stone in the middle containing the seed of the fruit;

much like that of a plum or peach), is a delicacy, prized across the world, not least for its delicious taste when ground up and made into the paste called marzipan. Its oil is one of the most favored by aromatherapists for use as a carrier for other oils. It is thin and light, and absorbs into the skin quickly, penetrating deeply into the tissues.

TRADITIONAL USES

There are two chemotypes, Bitter and Sweet Almond. Bitter almonds are rarely used as they contain a hydrogen cyanide, which is highly poisonous causing vertigo-like symptoms and in some cases even death. There is a Bitter Almond essential oil, which must be used in minuscule diluted amounts of less than 1%, where the poison is used to cleanse the system of parasites, intestinal worms and high fever.

MEDICINAL USES

Almond oil used as a carrier oil is highly antioxidant and nourishes the body with Vitamins A, B, and E. Almond is also good for helping the liver to detoxify and is beneficial for vascular complaints such as spider veins or varicose veins.

It has emollient properties meaning it traps moisture, helping to reduce dry and flaky skin. It has a light, sweet taste making it an excellent choice for making lip balms. When ground, the nuts make a wonderful facial scrub, clearing away dead cells and debris.

Bitter Almond should not be used during pregnancy and is recommended only be used at no more than 1% dilution as a compress to reduce fever and an abdominal massage treatment to expel intestinal worms. Sweet Almond is generally regarded as safe for all ages. Despite the fact that almond is not a nut, it could, however, cause an allergic reaction for nut allergy sufferers.

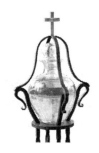

Anise

There is only one reference to Anise in the Bible. These few words alone show the importance of the seed during biblical times. In Matthew 23:23, it says:

> Woe unto you, scribes and Pharisees, hypocrites! For ye pay tithe of Mint and Anise and Cumin and have omitted the weightier matters of the law, judgment, mercy, and faith: these ought ye to have done, and not to leave the other undone.

Later translations argued the word Anise is better translated as Dill as used in the English Standard Version. Its honorable mention in such a weighty book has caused much conspiracy throughout the Church, regarding the tithe.

The law of tithing dictated that 10% of all crops and livestock must be given to the tabernacle. While it is only mentioned twice in the New Testament, it is recorded many times throughout the Old.

When you collect the information of Leviticus 27:30, Numbers 18:26, Deuteronomy 14:24 and 2 Chronicles 31:5, the tithing responsibility seems to grow like a seed. Gathering their responsibilities for agriculture, the poor, and the use of the temple for feasts, a Pharisee was expected to give a massive 23.3% in tithes. Later in the New Testament (according to Jesus' remarks rather than the Old Testament law), it was established that tithing should be according to a person's ability, how much they could afford and what was in their heart. This may be 10%, but it may be all as in the widow's mite. This key verse illustrates the change in attitude and expectation in the New Covenant.

As an extremely erudite and eloquent man, Yeshua's choice of spices would not have been accidental. He deliberately picked examples that would make the biggest impact. The fact that he chose Anise to flatter the Pharisees on their devout reverence for the tithing law only to scorn their lack of judgment and reverence to God shows Anise must have been tithed in vast amounts. In other words, in contrast, you give so much of the easy stuff, but when it comes to hard substance from your core, you deliver so little.

Anise was in good supply and widely available during ancient times. There are records in ancient Egyptian literature showing it grew as a common herb throughout Syria, Egypt, and the Levant. The herb also grew wild in many parts and was extremely easy to cultivate.

Dioscorides (A.D. 40-90) wrote that Anise induces sexual desire and also states that Pythagoras (570-495 B.C.) favored Anise to treat scorpion stings. Two thousand years before, the ancient Egyptians frequently placed Anise flowers along with Cumin and Marjoram into the emptied cadaver to scent it prior to mummification. Perhaps there was more than purely the aroma evoked by this, as Anise is mentioned medicinally in papyri for their digestive prowess. In Papyrus Ebers dating back to 1550 B.C., the reader is told to drink Anise to alleviate pain. Later in Papyrus Hearst, the hieroglyphs were translated to say Anise was a "gas banisher."

This digestive element coupled with its slightly risqué aphrodisiac dimension has made Anise (or sometimes written as Anise Seed) the base for many alcoholic beverages, including ouzo, pastis, and, of course, the legendary absinthe, which was banned in America in 1912 and many parts of Europe in 1915 because of its alleged hallucinogenic properties. The lesser known Anisette is placed on the head in a voodoo ritual to ward off the stare of the evil eye.

The first introduction of Anise to Europe and England was during the 14th century. Most likely it was brought by the Crusaders in the previous century. Interestingly, in 1305 Edward I once again pledged a tax on Anise to fund the repairs on London Bridge.

BIBLICAL REFERENCES TO ANISE

Matthew 23:23

ANISE'S HEALING PROPERTIES

The sweet, fragrant scent of Anise has been popular since ancient times when it was commonly used in herbal medicine to treat digestive complaints. It is a pretty herb, and a distant relative to the carrot. Belonging to the Apiaceae family, it grows to around a foot in height, has light wispy leaves and flowers prolifically through June until August with white or yellow flowers depending on its strain.

Native to Greece and Egypt, Anise essential oil is steam distilled from the seeds of the plant. For blending in aromatherapy, Anise essential oil is a top note. Its aroma is rich and sweet, with an Aniseed-like fragrance that is instantly recognizable.

Anise is comprised of 90% anethole, which is responsible for its distinctive aroma. It is often confused with Star Anise, which belongs to a different family but has a similar fragrance and chemical composition. The warm, sweet scent of Anise blends well with other spice oils, including Cardamom, Caraway, Cedarwood, Coriander, Dill, Fennel, Mandarin, Petitgrain, and Rosewood.

TRADITIONAL USES

As a sweetly spicy herb, Anise was also in very high demand in biblical times. Throughout ancient literature Anise is mentioned over and over again for its stomachic uses. By far, its most famous use was like a precursor to toothpaste. The pungent taste and flavor freshened breath as well as aided digestion.

In ancient times, Anise was also added to potpourri to protect the household from evil spirits or the "evil eye." Placing Anise beneath your pillow was also thought to prevent nightmares.

In biblical times, Anise was used as a form of currency – as mentioned in Matthew 23:23, *Ye pay tithe of Mint, Anise, and Cumin.*

The Romans used Anise in their festive cake *mustaceae*. The digestive properties of Anise were recognized by the ancient Romans, who referred to the herb as *solamen intestinorum*, or "the comforter of the bowels." After a lavish wedding feast, this delicious spiced cake was served at the end of every festive occasion to aid digestion and prevent indigestion from the rich foods. Food historians believe the wedding cake recipe we recognize today initially stemmed from this early tradition.

MEDICINAL USES

Anise can help with a range of digestive complaints, including flatulence, constipation, indigestion, stomach gas, colic and intestinal worms. Its estrogenic properties can ease menstrual cramps, promote the production of breast milk and help to stimulate menstruation.

Its calming aroma can soothe anxiety, stress, depression and anger. Anise is also used for muscular aches and pains, spasms, bronchitis, coughs, colds, congestion, epileptic seizures, hysteria, vertigo, and migraines. As an antiseptic, it can be used to treat wounds and head lice.

Since biblical times, Anise has been used as a domestic spice and flavoring for food and beverages. It was also traditionally used to aid digestion and freshen the breath. Today, it is widely utilized in the pharmaceutical industry as a fragrance and/or flavoring for cough mixtures, lozenges, and dental products. In aromatherapy, it is most commonly used for digestive and respiratory ailments.

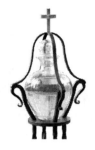

Balsam

Balsam comes from the sap of the tree *Commiphora opobalsamum*, also known as *Commiphora gildiensis*. It is referred to many times throughout the Old Testament by various names. It is called *bosem*, *besem*, and *nataf*. In the Talmud and Septuagint, it is referred to as *kataf*, *balsam*, *appobalsam* and *afarsemon*. *Afarsemon* is translated as Persimmon, and you will sometimes see the balsam groves referred to as persimmon groves. The persimmon, however, is from a different family. *Commiphora* is usually spiny trees that always secrete a sap.

In some passages of the Bible, *bosem* becomes synonymous with the term "perfume spices." However, for the most part, *bosem* was considered the **Balm of Gilead,** also known as the Balm of Mecca.

The first time Balsam is mentioned in the book of Genesis was when Joseph was betrayed by his brothers and cast down into a pit. As he lay there, his brothers feasted on their lunch. It says in Genesis 37:25:

> *As they sat down to eat their meal, they looked up and saw a caravan of Ishmaelites coming from Gilead. Their camels were loaded with spices, balm, and Myrrh, and they were on their way to take them down to Egypt.*

A merchant's bounty indeed. But what was the balm used for?

Later in the Old Testament, Jeremiah laments for his people, weeping that even the Balm of Gilead cannot be a salve for his loss. In Jeremiah 8:21-22 it states,

> *For the brokenness of the daughter of my people I am broken; I mourn, dismay has taken hold of me. Is there no balm in Gilead? Is there no physician there? Why then has not the health of the daughter of my people been restored?*

Medicine, we know, but for what? Many scholars believe it may have been an ingredient by another name called *stacte*, a vital component of the *ketoret*, the most sacred incense burned the tabernacles. The word stacte is translated as *nataf* in the Septuagint, which means "drop."

The sacred recipe for *ketoret* was given to Moses by God in Exodus 30:34-38 and 37:29,

> *And the LORD said unto Moses, Take unto yourself sweet spices, stacte, and onycha, and galbanum; these sweet spices with pure Frankincense: of each shall there be a like weight: And you shall make it a perfume, a confection after the art of the apothecary, tempered together [salted], pure and holy: And you shall beat some of it very small, and put of it before the testimony in the tabernacle of the congregation, where I will meet with you: it shall be unto you most holy. And as for the perfume which you shall make, you shall not make to yourselves according to the composition thereof: it shall be unto you holy for the LORD. Whosoever shall make like unto it, to enjoy the smell thereof, shall even be cut off from his people.*

The Holy Incense was burned twice daily on an altar made of Acacia wood and inlayed with beaten gold inside of the Golden Temple. On the holiest day, Yom Kippur, the Cohanim (priests) would draw the curtain back inside of the temple and burn *ketoret* on the altar inside of the Holy of Holies. The name *ketoret* means "to bond." Could Jeremiah's lament be a wish for a renewal of his bond?

To understand just how treasured this incense was, one needs to consider the ritual with Yahweh (God) and how the priests delivered it. Animal sacrifice signified the subjugation of man's basest urges and instincts, in an attempt to rid them from God's people. The creature would be caught and herded to the temple, kept there, slaughtered, cleaned, then burned. The stench of death in the heat would have been horrendous. The ketoret not only separated the priests from the stench and effectively made them clean from it, but also transcended them above the human urges. The environment was cleansed and the garments made fresh; in so doing God's people were lifted closer to him.

It has been said the fragrance was so pungent, ladies as far away as Jericho had no need to wear perfume as the incense filled the air.

The tree *commipora opobalsamum* is extremely hard to cultivate, and so the trees are very rare. In Turkey, they are so protected there is a ban on importation of the plant. The writings of Josephus tell us the Queen of Sheba took the balm of Gilead as a gift to charm Solomon, which might indicate the scarcity that may have always existed.

Dioscorides describes *opobalsam* as "juice flowing from the balsam tree." The small tree grows to around 12 feet in height and spontaneously exudes a sap in the heat. Incisions are slashed into its reddish bark so the juice can flow out. The essential oil makes up around one-quarter of the juice content. This unguent flow or repeated "drop" is what persuades scholars the balm is probably the *stacte* in the incense recipe.

Moslem and Coptic lore both tell a tale of Mary visiting a garden in Ayn Shams in Egypt and washing Christ's clothes in the water. By the Middle Ages, Ayn Shams was the only place where the *Communis opobalsamum* would grow. It is said it was because the water Christ had charmed must touch its source.

Balsam is the only tropical and most expensive spice grown naturally in Israel. From the balm grew a famous and extremely lucrative perfumery business. Its delicious lemony vanilla scent makes it an instant hit with the ladies and it is said many royal ladies wore its fragrance. Around the prosperous groves of Ein Gedi, a massive religious center, a thriving economy grew around this ointment.

Josephus' records indicate that tensions were at their highest between Cleopatra and Herod the Great, in which Cleopatra contemplated seducing Herod to antagonize her husband, Mark Anthony. On consideration, she discovered a far more powerful play and encouraged Mark Anthony to give her the Balsam Groves at Ein Gedi. The title deeds were handed over to the queen, issuing a fierce blow to Israel.

After Cleopatra's death, Herod leased the groves back, and the economy started to strengthen again. However, peace was short-lived because the temptation of the Balm of Gilead now had Rome in its grasp.

During the times of Roman occupation, curtailing their chances of income was an extremely useful strategy. Pliny often speaks of the plant in his *Historia Naturalis* and tells how Vespasian had wanted to bring the Balm back to Rome. This triggered a dangerous fascination in his son Titus who became determined to capture the precious Balsam orchards.

The Jews fiercely protected their Balsam orchards for many years, but Titus was finally able to seize them. In his victory march to Rome, Titus displayed many Balsam trees he had captured from Judea. Later the Balsam collected from those orchards was to become one of Rome's most important sources of income. Titus later became the first son to succeed his father to the throne of Emperor. Balsam, no doubt, played a pivotal role in his campaign.

Control of the Balsam plantations stayed under royal control, and the methods of extraction were a carefully guarded secret. During the 2nd century, Jewish fighters determined to curtail the progress of Rome uprooted the trees to prevent Rome from having them. Bar Kokhba Revolt was one of the most famous turning points in the Jewish wars.

Ein Gedi is still today an oasis, flourishing with flora and fauna. It takes its name from "spring of the goat kid," after the ibex who wander over its lands. Balsam, though, has been absent for many centuries. In the 7th century, Muslims overtook the country and flooded it with cheaper perfumes. The allure of the Balsam was gone.

Since 2010, horticulturalists have been painstakingly trying to raise new *Commiphora opobalsamum* plants on the banks at Ein Gedi. A failed attempt to restore the plant in the 1970s dashed hopes of the groves being restored. In the 1990s, seeds from Ethiopia and the Sudan were planted, but again *Commiphora opobalsamum* refused to grow. Then in 2003, Dr. Michael Avishai brought seeds from England from which saplings had been raised. In 2010, after an absence of 2,000 years, the Balsam returned home to Ein Gedi.

BIBLICAL REFERENCES TO BALSAM

2 Samuel 5:23
2 Samuel 5:24
1 Chronicles 14:14
1 Chronicles 14:15

BALSAM'S HEALING PROPERTIES

In biblical times, a healing substance known as Balm of Gilead was made from the resin of the *Commiphora opobalsamum* bush, which was native to the area of Gilead.

The healing property of Balm of Gilead, also known as Balm of Mecca, is mentioned several times in the Bible. Balsam was expensive, highly prized and used as a form of currency. It is believed that Balsam was among the gifts presented to King Solomon by the Queen of Sheba. The deep, warm aroma of Balsam made it an attractive perfume in ancient times.

Commiphora opobalsamum belongs to the Burseraceae family and is native to countries surrounding both sides of the Red Sea – including Egypt, Ethiopia, Saudi Arabia and Sudan.

Balsam is extracted from the resinous juice of the plant. During the summer, the white resin oozes out from the trunk and gradually turns grey and solid when exposed to the air.

Its potent aroma has a woody, oily, balsamic tone. For aromatherapy blending, it is classed as a base note. Balsam combines well with other woody oils such as Pine, Cedarwood, Benzoin, Lavender, Spruce, Frankincense, Lemon and Rosemary.

The chemical constituents of Balsam include compounds that resemble salicylates, found in aspirin, which is an effective analgesic and anti-inflammatory.

TRADITIONAL USES

Balsam was traditionally used as a healing salve for bites and wounds, as well as for treating respiratory conditions and headaches. Its miraculous healing properties were highly venerated, to the extent it was once believed that a finger coated with Balsam was completely protected from fire. As a natural pain-reliever, Balsam was also massaged into areas of rheumatism, aches, and sprains.

MEDICINAL USES

For thousands of years, Balsam has been used to heal skin disorders such as bites, sores, wounds, eczema, and ulcers. It eases digestive complaints and fight infections, colds, and fever. Balsam also affects the reproductive system by boosting fertility.

Balsam is useful for lowering blood pressure due to its naturally hypotensive properties. Studies have shown that Balm of Gilead also may have an anti-cancerous effect on tumor cells. Its antimicrobial qualities are effective against bacteria, including Staphylococcus aureus.

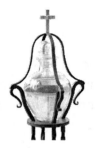

Bay Laurel

Laurel Nobilis is an evergreen tree that can grow to a towering height of 70 feet. Its pale yellow leaves are born in pairs along its glossy green leaves. The Laurel is a dioecious tree meaning it is unisexual having male and female flowers growing on separate plants.

The Bay Laurel is a very hardy tree that grows around the Mediterranean and in Israel in most environments. Thriving in sand, loam and clay, the Bay Laurel came to be synonymous to the Israelites with victory, honor, and flourishing. Years after the Israelite nation survived regardless of famine and wars, they began to associate the Laurel tree with their homeland, which had reached a height of development and influence.

There is only one direct mention of the tree in the Bible's Old Testament, but in the New Testament, it becomes an oft-used symbol through the Epistles. Psalm 37, most likely written by King David in his latter days, describes how he mourns over the wicked who seem to prosper so easily. In the New Living translation, it says in Psalm 37:35,

> *I have seen wicked and ruthless people flourishing like a tree in its native soil.*

Moreover, in the English Standard Version, it reads, *I have seen a wicked, ruthless man, spreading himself like a green laurel tree.*

The flourishing Laurel tree tends to grow large with numerous branches, spreading its canopy regardless of what type of soil it is in. Only two things might upset it. In the desert heat, its leaves may go brown, or if it is transplanted, it may suffer some stress.

The two translations here cover both aspects. The wicked man has not had to undergo transplantation. Therefore, his roots are dug firm into the ground, and nothing seems to faze him as he prospers and boasts of his success. In this comparison, the Laurel tree depicts both prosperity and fame. But, the King exhorts his people not be tempted or fooled by the ways of the wicked.

Later the Psalm describes how the King returned, but this time, the wicked had vanished. While the wicked may enjoy brief success in their accomplishments, God's enemies are like grass and quickly fade away. Here the psalmist compares the Bay Laurel to God's continual sustained help to the righteous. God will always be there for you and uphold you even in unbearable conditions.

In the New Testament, the use of the Laurel is implied by the term "crown," which is mainly utilized by the Apostle Paul. Paul, who had been very heavily influenced by the Greek and Roman culture, depicts the Laurel as an image of triumph and excellence. After a battle, the Roman battalions sent a bay wreath ahead of them to the emperor to convey they had been victorious.

On four separate occasions, Paul invokes the image of a Laurel crown as a metaphor for excellence in ushering in the Kingdom of Heaven. In 1 Peter 5:4 NIV it says,

> *And when the chief Shepherd shall appear,*
> *ye shall receive a crown of glory that*
> *fadeth not away.*

As an athletic trainer who must endure strict training to receive the medal or trophy, so here St. Paul alludes to the Isthmian games, well known to the Corinthians. Those who were steadfast in their conviction to win the games would survive on very lean diets and work extremely hard to become fit.

Of course, the leaf crown would not last, but believers are encouraged to exercise their faith and compete for the crown that will last forever. He uses the Laurel crown as a metaphor for the prize given to those who gave up carnal pursuits and renounced sin. Similarly, anyone who competes as an athlete does not receive the victor's crown except by competing according to the rules.

A favorite passage of Scripture for many is Paul's beautifully poignant final letter to St. Timothy, where he is clearly well aware of the nearness of the end of his life. He welcomes it, comforted by the conviction he has trained and run his course. In 2 Timothy 4:7 KJV it reads,

> *I have fought the good fight, I have finished the course, I have kept the faith; in the future there is laid up for me the crown of righteousness, which the Lord, the righteous Judge, will award to me on that day; and not only to me, but also to all who have loved His appearing.*

In every instance, a reference to the most glorious thing he can think of, such as the Laurel victor's crown, it is trumped by the salvation of the eternal crown of Christ.

BIBLICAL REFERENCES TO BAY LAUREL

Psalm 37:35
Isaiah 44:14

SPICE CHEST: VICTORY OVER SIN

In St. Paul's Cathedral, a beautifully carved laurel wreath represents Christ's victory over sin. Even death, which held no dominion over him, was sealed by his resurrection with an everlasting crown of evergreen leaves.

Laurel was believed to have supernatural powers to protect people from misfortune and in biblical times, it was customary to plant a Bay Laurel close to the house to deter lightning. Bay Laurel leaves were believed to give oracles and soothsayers the ability to see into the future. Roman Emperors exploited this trait to the fullest; Tiberius was terrified of lightening and so is reputed to have slept completely naked except for a Laurel nightcap. Nero followed suit by insisting at every meeting he had to be convened beneath a Laurel tree.

Interestingly, the Bay still carries the significance of triumph and excellence. French students pass their baccalaureate, which takes its name from "berries of the bay." Still others celebrate poetic brilliance with bay, the poet laureate.

BAY LAUREL'S HEALING PROPERTIES

Bay Laurel, a popular culinary herb, belongs to the Lauraceae family, one of the largest botanical groups of woody trees and shrubs. Native to the Mediterranean region, Bay Laurel has been used since ancient times for both medicinal and culinary purposes. Nowadays, Bay Laurel is still widely used as a fragrance and flavoring agent in a range of toiletries, perfumes, drinks and processed foods. The tree is also called the True Laurel and Sweet Bay Laurel, with its leaves popularly used as a culinary seasoning.

Bay Laurel essential oil is steam distilled from the leaves and branches of the tree. As a top note, it has a spicy, medicinal aroma that blends well with Pine, Cypress, Juniper, Rosemary, Clary Sage, Lavender and spice oils. Cineol (also known as eucalyptol) constitutes around half the chemical composition of Bay Laurel oil, which explains the camphor-like element to its fragrance.

TRADITIONAL USES

In biblical times, Bay Laurel symbolized prominence, fame, and affluence. The ancient Greeks believed it to have divine powers, with the ability to ward off thunder, lightning, evil and disease. Its leaves were woven into garlands and crowns to represent victory. Herbalists traditionally used Bay Laurel to treat a variety of respiratory and digestive problems.

MEDICINAL USES

The digestive properties of Bay Laurel make it an excellent herb for treating dyspepsia, flatulence, and loss of appetite. It can also help respiratory conditions, such as colds, flu, tonsillitis and viral infections. As an emmenagogue, Bay Laurel can help to regulate absent or scanty periods. It encourages the elimination of excess fluid and wastes by promoting increased sweating and urination.

Other medicinal uses of Bay Laurel include the treatment of arthritis, rheumatism, headaches, bruises and high blood pressure. Scientific studies have shown that Bay Laurel can inhibit melanoma (a form of skin cancer) cell proliferation at high concentrations. Modern research also indicates that Bay Laurel may have the ability to regulate insulin levels in the body.

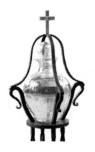

Bdellium

The Bdellium of the Bible seems to come from a tree closely related to Myrrh's *Commiphora africana*. *Commiphora africana* (A.Rich.) is commonly referred to as African Myrrh. It is a small deciduous tree belonging to the Burseraceae. It occurs widely over sub-Saharan Africa in Angola, Botswana, Burkina Faso, Chad, Eritrea, Ethiopia, Kenya, Mali, Mauritania, Mozambique, Namibia, Niger, Senegal, Somalia, South Africa, Sudan, Swaziland, Tanzania, Uganda, Zambia, and Zimbabwe.

This tree grows best in very sandy environments. It will grow to 5 meters (about 16 feet) high and has long spiny branches. Its peeling, grey-green bark splits and reveals lustrous red wood, which oozes Bdellian sap when the sun hits it. At the first touch of spring, the wood bursts into bright green leaves. These leaves remain bright and vivid throughout the rainy season. Then, it bares small red berries about 6-8 millimeters across which provides abundant nutrition for the local birds. The sap is collected and dried and is believed to be the treasured Bdellium of the Bible.

It is mentioned in two ways in the Bible. The first mention of it comes in Genesis 2:12. In Genesis 2:12 we see an excellent example of how the books were constructed to lay reverence at the doorway of Yahweh. In Genesis 2:11-13 NASB it reads,

> *The name of the first is Pishon; it flows around the whole land of Havilah, where there is gold. The gold of that land is good; the bdellium and the onyx stone are there. The name of the second river is Gihon; it flows around the whole land of Cush.*

Consider the lush green paradise of Eden, every branch laden with her bounty, but Adam and Eve in their wisdom disobeyed God and were cast out of the garden. Always after would their descendants struggle. Here we see the description of the place they must go. No greenery and laden trees are described here. Instead, minerals and incenses they know they can trade. Now they must work for their living. This verse symbolizes man's separation from God.

Bible commentators disagree here whether the verse does, in fact, pertain to the resin because the resin is at odds with the precious metal and stone. Many assert the word is better translated as "pearls." Later, however, the names of Bdellium do arise again, but this time, by its Hebrew name *Bedolach* and the translation here seems sound to be listed as Bdellium.

The scriptures tell us the Hebrews complained about their manna, which tasted like Coriander seed and its appearance was like that of Bdellium in Numbers 11:7.

This well-loved ingredient in Biblical times was a beautifully scented resin that softened and seeped from the *Commiphora africana* on warm days helped by incisions into the bark. Its distinctive scent was frequently worn by ancient Egyptian ladies as perfume.

Because of it being a relatively cheap ingredient, it was often used to adulterate its more costly cousin, Myrrh.

In A.D. 200 Galen wrote in his work *On Antidotes* of having read an essay by Damocrates (A.D. 50) where he cites Rufus of Ephesus using Bdellium to make the sacred Egyptian incense *kyphi*. The papyrus explained how the incense was used to purify the temple and could also be used as an antidote for snakebites.

To create the great *kyphi*, Rufus relates, "Honey and raisins should be mashed together well. Bdellium and Myrrh should be ground with some wine until the mixture has the consistency of runny honey. Then it should be combined with the honey and raisin mixture.

Other ingredients, Frankincense, Cardamom, and Myrrh, were ground and added, and the incense was then shaped into pellets for burning."

Some other ancient sources describe Bdellium, which offers insight into its uses. The Greek philosopher Theophastrus, who succeeded Aristotle in the Peripatetic school and was considered to be "The Father of Plants" because of his many botanical works, is one of the earliest references we have to the plant (dated c. 371 – c. 287 B.C.).

He writes, "In the region called Aria there is a thorn tree which produces a tear of resin, resembling Myrrh in appearance and odor. It liquefies when the sun shines upon it."

Pliny the Elder describes the best Bdellium coming from Bactria as a "tree black in color and the size of the Olive tree; its leaf resembles that of the oak and its fruit the wild fig." Compare that with the claims of Isidore of Seville in his Etymologiae (XVII.viii.6) that "Bdellium comes from trees in India and Arabia, the Arabian variety being better as it is smooth, whitish and smells good; the Indian variety is a dirty black."

We know, too, from the Periplus of the Erythraean Sea, (c. A.D. 200), Bdella were exported from the port of Barbarice at the mouth of the Indus.

BIBLICAL REFERENCES TO BDELLIUM

Genesis 2:12
Numbers 11:7

BDELLIUM'S HEALING PROPERTIES

Bdellium is a type of resin extracted by steam distillation from the *Commiphora africana* tree, which is commonly known as African Myrrh. All parts of the plant have traditionally been used for medicinal and perfumery purposes.

With a bitter, spicy fragrance that is very similar to Myrrh, Bdellium is often substituted as a cheaper alternative to the real thing. Both belong to the Burseraceae family of flowering plants. Like Myrrh, Bdellium is a base note that blends well with Benzoin, Frankincense, Lavender, Sandalwood, Clove, and Patchouli.

TRADITIONAL USES

The ancient Greek Theophrastus was one of the first to write about Bdellium, which was described as "resembling Myrrh in appearance and odor" in his classic text *Enquiry into Plants*. In ancient Egypt, Bdellium was used as a perfume and carried in small pouches by Egyptian women. Since then, Bdellium has traditionally been used as an insecticide, aphrodisiac, and treatment for skin problems.

In the Bible, Bdellium is mentioned in the depiction of the Garden of Eden, and the land of Havilah *where there is gold; and the gold of that land is good: there is Bdellium and the onyx stone* (Genesis 2:11). Manna is compared to Bdellium, indicating that the plant was highly prized by the Hebrews.

MEDICINAL USES

The resin of Bdellium is used to treat digestive disorders, including diarrhea, indigestion, flatulence and loss of appetite. Its fragrance is emotionally balancing, which soothes stress and helps to induce sleep. Bdellium is a useful remedy for arthritis and menstrual problems, as well as respiratory conditions including coughs, colds, catarrh, asthma and sore throats. It is also known for its use as a skin treatment, for everything from acne to wounds, fungal infections, sores, aging skin and sun damage.

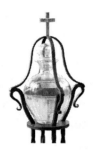

Calamus

Calamus Root, also known as Sweet Flag, was well known in biblical times and mentioned in Exodus 30:22-25 as one of the ingredients of the Holy Anointing Oil. Calamus is also listed as a chief principle spice in the Song of Solomon and mentioned in the book of Ezekiel. For thousands of years, Calamus has been an item of trade in many cultures for its wide variety of medicinal uses, and it value in the perfume industry. This herb has traditionally been smoked, eaten, or brewed into a tea, decoction, extract, tincture and syrup. According to Ayurvedic tradition, Vacha is a 'sattvic' herb, which feeds and transmutes the sexual 'kundalini' energy. Calamus has been called "the closest thing to a sex stimulant that nature has to offer." *Acorus Calamus* was also used by the ancient Greeks and included in the traditional remedies of many other European cultures.

In Britain, the plant was cut for use as a sweet smelling floor covering for packed earth floors of medieval dwellings and churches, and stacks of rushes were used as the centerpiece of rush bearing ceremonies for many hundreds of years. It was also used as a thatching material for English cottages. In antiquity in the Orient and Egypt, the rhizome was thought to be a powerful aphrodisiac. In Europe, *Acorus calamus* was often added to wine, with its root one of the possible ingredients of absinthe. Among the northern Native Americans, it is used both medicinally and as a stimulant.

The word "Calamus" in Hebrew is *Qaneh*, which means "a stalk or aromatic reed." It is translated as "right or upright," "balances" and "measuring rod" in Scripture. The first biblical example of the word to mean "moral uprightness" in Exodus 15:26 says, *Do that which is right in his sight.*

Calamus is a reminder of how Yeshua is upright and righteous in his Father's eyes, an example we should follow. 2 Corinthians 5:21 tells us,

> *For he hath made him [to be] sin for us,*
> *who knew no sin; that we might be made*
> *the righteousness of God in him.*

The Scriptures tell us Yahweh searches to and fro for those who are upright. 2 Chronicles 16:9 says:

For the eyes of the LORD run to and fro throughout the whole earth, to show himself strong in the behalf of [them] whose heart [is] perfect toward him. Herein thou hast done foolishly: therefore, from henceforth thou shalt have wars.

BIBLICAL REFERENCES TO CALAMUS

Exodus 30:23
Song of Solomon 4:14
Ezekiel 27:19

CALAMUS' HEALING PROPERTIES

Calamus essential oil is extracted from the perennial Calamus Root, which grows to a height of 1 meter (about 3 feet). Its name is derived from a Greek term for "reed," which represents its rush-like appearance. Calamus is sometimes known as "Sweet Flag," along with several other aliases. The rhizome is horizontal, creeping, cylindrical, branched and up to 2 meters long (around 6.5 feet), with a spicy aroma; the fruit is greenish berries. Indigenous to the northern hemisphere, it prefers lake margins, swampy ditches, or marshes in a protected position. It is frost resistant, but drought tender.

Native to India, Calamus belongs to the Acoraceae family. Its essential oil is extracted from the rhizomes by steam distillation. As a base note, it brings a deep, refreshing scent that is akin to Cinnamon. In aromatherapy, it blends well with Lavender, Tea Tree, Rosemary, Clary Sage, Geranium, and Marjoram.

TRADITIONAL USES

For thousands of years, *Acorus calamus* has been used as a traditional remedy for a broad range of conditions including nervous disorders, loss of appetite, respiratory infections, skin diseases and digestive problems. There is evidence of its use dating back to ancient Egyptian times when traces of Calamus were found in Tutankhamen's tomb.

The plant was also used as an herbal remedy in Europe throughout the Middle Ages. It was most commonly used to help calm the mind, ward off evil, clear phlegm and congestion, and aid in digestion. Traditionally, Calamus was drunk as an herbal tea, although oral ingestion is no longer recommended due to its potential toxicity.

MEDICINAL USES

Calamus essential oil is used to provide relief from muscular spasms, rheumatism, gout, and arthritis. It can stimulate the brain and nervous system, helping to balance mental disorders such as memory loss and shock. Its ability to repair damaged brain tissues and neurons can contribute to treating neuralgia, nervous afflictions, and epilepsy. It helps to contract blood vessels to reduce pressure on the cranial nerve, which relieves pain from neuralgia and headaches. As an antirheumatic and anti-arthritic oil, Calamus is known to stimulates the nervous system. It is also known to stimulate metabolism.

As a circulation booster, Calamus encourages the flow of oxygen and nutrients around the body, which in turn helps to stimulate the metabolism. Studies on rats have proven it to have a neuroprotective effect against strokes and neurodegeneration. It also protects against acrylamide-induced neurotoxicity.

Due to its toxicity, Calamus can be used as an effective antioxidant to treat internal and external infections, as they cannot survive in its presence. It also does not allow any biotic growth and acts an antibiotic, which is useful for fighting infections.

Calamus essential oil is known for its antispasmodic properties and is good for treating spasms. It is recommended this oil be used in very mild doses for nervous conditions. This oil is a nervive, aiding in maintaining good health for the nervous system. It reduces the occurrence of an epileptic attack. Because of this oil's effect on the brain, it supports the memory, which is beneficial to those who have memory loss due to aging, trauma or disease. Calamus can help repair the damage done to the brain tissues and neurons.

When used in moderation, Calamus can help to calm the mind, promote positive thoughts, and relax the body. In very low doses it can induce sleep and work as a tranquilizer for those who suffer from insomnia or sleeplessness. Further, due to its numbing and tranquilizing effect on the brain and the nerves, it reduces the feeling of pain. This oil may be used for the treatment of a headache, vertigo, or as a sedative.

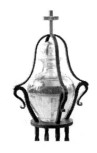

Cassia

Cassia is mentioned in Exodus 30:22-31 as part of the Holy Anointing Oil. The Hebrew word for the spice Cassia is similar to the word meaning "to bow down or to pay homage." The word homage in the Scriptures means "to honor another by bending low with profound respect." Yeshua's Bride is to be humble toward all people. She is to bow down in homage to God alone.

Cassia and Cinnamon are very similar in fragrance because they are actually of the same genus and Laurel family of plants. Cassia was considered inferior to other plants in the Laurel family, according to the Department of Agriculture.

Isn't that true of Yeshua's life? Yeshua said, *I honor My Father... I seek not mine own glory* in John 8:49-50.

Like Cassia, Yeshua was considered lowly and honored the Father in everything he did. The leaders considered him of little account because he came from Nazareth, but his Father glorified him as mentioned in John 8:54: *Jesus answered, If I honor myself, my honor is nothing: it is my Father that honoureth me; of whom ye say, that he is your God.*

In the Middle Ages, the Arabs maintained a monopoly of the spice trade by claiming Cinnamon and/or Cassia was harvested from the nests of ferocious birds and had to be gathered under their attack.

In both Hebrew and Arabic, the root word *Kiddah* signifies "a strip," referring to the strips of bark from which the spice is made. In addition to honoring and bending down to pay homage, Cassia spiritually speaks of being stripped of arrogance and pride and walking in humility with a servant's heart and attitude. This is also one of the fragrances mentioned in Psalm 45:8 that Yeshua's garments are soaked in.

Cassia is one of the principle spices in the Holy Anointing Oil and was commonly traded along the incense trail. Cassia was used in the anointing oil to anoint priests, kings, and their garments. Likewise, the coming King Messiah's robes will smell of Cassia.

In the spiritual sense, Cassia speaks of humility, being stripped of pride, set apart as holy with a servant's heart.

The deep, exotic aroma and the rich color of our new Cassia oil make it a welcome addition to our family of biblical fragrant anointing oils. Psalm 45:8 says, *Your robes are all fragrant with Myrrh, Aloes, and Cassia...*

BIBLICAL REFERENCES TO CASSIA

Exodus 30:24
Ezekiel 27:19
Psalm 45:8

SPICE CHEST: HONOR TO THE FATHER ALONE

Cassia, though considered an inferior plant to the other species in the Laurel family, is mentioned in the book of Exodus as part of the Holy Anointing Oil. The Hebrew word for "Cassia" is *Qiddah*, which is similar to the word meaning "to bow down" or "to pay homage." "Homage" in Scripture means to honor another by bending low in profound respect. As his bride and as Yeshua did, we are to bow down in homage to the Heavenly Father alone.

CASSIA'S HEALING PROPERTIES

Cinnammomum cassia is indigenous to China and is known as the Chinese Cinnamon, which they used extensively in their medicine. It was introduced into Europe during classical times by Arabian and Phoenician traders. Cassia or *"kwei"* in early Chinese herbal by Shen-nung, is the spice sold in the United States as Cinnamon. Cinnamon Bark (*Cinnamomum zeylanicum*) from Ceylon is the true Cinnamon. The two are similar, but the Cinnamon has a sweeter, more delicate taste. Both contain cinamic aldehyde as their main component with Cassia having a greater concentration.

Cinnamomum cassia is an evergreen tree growing to up to 20 feet tall with a white aromatic bark and angular branches. The leaves are oblong-lanceolate about 18 centimeters (7 inches) long. Small yellow flowers hang from long stocks, and bloom in early summer. Cassia grows in hot, wet, tropical climates both wild and commercially. Once the tree reaches maturity, the stems are cut down. The bark is removed in short lengths and dried, with some varieties rolling into quills.

Most Cassia is ground into powder and sold under the label of Cinnamon. It can be distinguished from Cinnamon when it is sold in sticks. The Cinnamon is rolled into one roll or quill while Cassia is rolled from both sides giving the appearance of a scroll. The bark of the two herbs is similar in appearance but different in strength and quality. Cassia's outer bark is darker, thicker and coarser, but the inner bark is a smoother reddish brown.

The essential oil is coaxed from the bark by steam distilling it. The viscous pale-yellow to clear-red liquid has an intense aroma. Cassia is a dermal irritant and can redden the skin, so do not use directly on the skin without being diluted. It is best used aromatically.

Like its cousin Cinnamon, Cassia belongs to the Lauraceae botanical family. It is a favorite culinary spice, and often referred to as "Chinese Cinnamon." The essential oil is steam distilled from the leaves, bark, twigs and stalks of the evergreen tree, which is native to China. Its aroma is sweet, woody and spicy – a top note that blends well with many oils, including Benzoin, Clove Bud, Grapefruit, Lavender, Rosemary, Thyme and other spice oils.

TRADITIONAL USES

As one of the most antiseptic of all essential oils, Cassia has been traditionally used to treat all types of infections – particularly fungal infections, such as ringworm and Candida. In both Eastern and Western medicine, it has been used for thousands of years as a natural remedy for cataracts, atherosclerosis, dyspepsia, diarrhea, rheumatism, high blood pressure, kidney problems, colds, colic, and nausea. In ancient Chinese medicine, Cassia was commonly used to treat vascular conditions.

MEDICINAL USES

Cassia is extremely effective in fighting bacteria and viruses. Research has revealed that most viruses, fungi, and bacteria cannot sustain themselves in the presence of therapeutic quality essential oils such as Cassia and it was probably this oil that protected the Israelites from disease.

Cassia essential oil can be used as a tonic, carminative, and stimulant. It is used to treat nausea, flatulence, and diarrhea. Chinese and Japanese scientists have found that Cassia has sedative effects and lowers high blood pressure and fever in animal experiments. The oil has antiseptic properties, killing various types of bacteria and fungi. Cassia oil is used mainly as a carminative (for relieving colic and griping) or as a stomach tonic. It can also be used for colds, influenza, fevers, arthritis and rheumatism. Recent experiments in China have shown that Cassia can provide protection from radiation.

Cassia can be used to soothe dry, sensitive skin – as long as it is well diluted in carrier oil. It can be used to heal fungal nail infections, along with other infectious skin diseases. For digestive problems, Cassia can help to treat diarrhea, gas, nausea, vomiting and intestinal infections. As a stimulant, it helps to boost the circulation and will bring warmth and relief to stiff joints, rheumatism, and arthritis. It can also ease period pain and help to regulate the menstrual cycle. Cassia supports the immune system and is effective in fighting all types of bacterial and viral infections, including coughs, colds, flu and other respiratory conditions. Its sweet, uplifting aroma can improve mental wellbeing and aid depression. Its medicinal properties include being anti-inflammatory, antifungal, antibacterial, antiviral, and anticoagulant. Cassia helps to support the immune system and the body's natural defenses.

Benefits of Cassia oil include offering support to the immunity system against colds and flu simply by inhaling them or rubbing them on the soles of the feet. Cassia is being used to cure diabetes, high blood sugar, and high blood pressure according to the U.S. Department of Agriculture. It also calms spasms of the digestive tract, indigestion, diarrhea, colitis, vomiting, and nausea. This oil may also be used on the skin, but you should always dilute with a carrier oil such as Olive oil.

SPICE CHEST: THE SCENT OF HIS COMING

When Yeshua returns, the world will smell his coming! His garments will be scented with these biblical fragrances. Psalm 45:7-8 says:

> *Thou lovest righteousness, and hatest wickedness: therefore God, thy God, hath anointed thee with the oil of gladness above thy fellows. All thy garments smell of Myrrh, and Aloes, and Cassia, out of the ivory palaces, whereby they have made thee glad.*

These fragrances burn as incense before the throne of Yah and Yeshua's fragrance fills the Temple. Revelation 8:3-4 says,

> *And another angel came and stood at the altar, having a golden censer;*

and there was given unto him much incense, that he should offer it with the prayers of all saints upon the golden altar which was before the throne. And the smoke of the incense, which came with the prayers of the saints, ascended up before God out of the angel's hand.

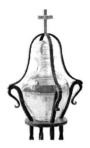

Cedarwood

His countenance is as Lebanon, excellent as the cedars,
Song of Solomon 5:15 tells us. The beloved Shulamite
intoned this canticle about her King, comparing his
presence to the stately trees residing in Lebanon.

Lebanon, the home of the Cedar, derives its name from
the root word *Leban* meaning "white." Its mountains,
blanketed with snow most of the year, provided the
necessary moisture to keep the trees thriving on its
slopes. Fed by melting streams of water, they yielded up
a fragrance that filled the valleys and covered the hills, a
fragrance of spiritual elevation. What a beautiful picture
of the remnant bride of Messiah, planted upon the
mountains in the Garden of God, elevated in the exalted

and heavenly places in Christ, filling the depressions and reaching the heights while continually offering up a fragrance that revealed their source of life.

Cedar is mentioned numerous times in the Bible, all in the Old Testament. For instance, in the beautiful Song of Songs in the Bible, the poetic description that begins, *My beloved is white and ruddy, the chiefest among ten thousands,* finishes with, *His countenance is as Lebanon, excellent as the cedars.*

Other references to Cedar include:

The cedar in the heaven of God is unmatched by Cypress and unresembling in its branches...

The trees of God resemble the Cedars of Lebanon which he planted.

The righteous flourish like the palm tree and grows like the cedar in Lebanon.

My love is white and red... bright as Lebanon and young as the cedars.

The scriptures in the book of Ezekiel illustrate beautifully how the noble kings of the forest were used by Prophet Orators to symbolize and typify worldly might, power, and glory. Thus, one obtains a fair idea of the crowning insolence of Sennacherib, the invader, when he boasted in the year 700 B.C. told of in 2 Kings 19:23,

> *I am come up the height of the mountains, to the sides of Lebanon; and I will cut down the tall cedars thereof.*

In J. Preston Eby's Kingdom Bible Studies entitled, *The Ashes of a Red Heifer*, he describes the fagots of cedar that are cast into the fire with Hyssop and scarlet as the burning heifer is consumed in the flames. As one of the ingredients of the water of separation, it is for the purification of defilement that is contracted by contact with death, symbolic of this world's system.

Eby writes, "The Cedar speaks to us of 'The Fragrance of His Life,' which, of course, is known only by exposing ourselves to His presence. The cedar tree has long stood as the symbol of eternal life and is also known predominately for its fragrance. Here is the picture of life bowing to the ravaging flames, but yielding up its glory at the same time, and imparting a fragrance to the sacrifice. The Cedar filled the mountains and the valleys with its delightful sacrifice, yielding up the fullness thereof in the final burst of perfume that the sacrifice might be acceptable to the nostril of God and efficacious for all to whom it is applied.

"One of the distinguishing characteristics of Lebanon was its smell. The fragrance that filled the valleys and covered the slopes of the mountains came from the most majestic of trees, Cedars. 'The smell of your garments is like the smell of Lebanon' (Song of Solomon 4:11). The smell of Lebanon was the smell of a tree, a tree that would yield its fragrance day after day, night after night, unchanging with the passing time. Summer and winter, in tropical heat or mountain cold, the cedar gave up the perfume for the garments of the King.

"The very name by which the tree was known, *EREZ* in Hebrew, means 'firmly rooted and strong.' It is a tree that has always been held in high esteem, not only for its vigor and beauty but also for its fragrance and the lasting quality of its wood. There is something permanent, something continuing about the scent of this tree. Shrubs that bloomed give up their odors for a time, but then the flowers fade and wither away, and the fragrance is no more. Annuals bloom for a while, perhaps a day or a week, but then they too, fade away, and the sweet smell becomes just a memory of yesterday. Not so the odor of the cedar tree, especially the Cedars of Lebanon. The fragrance of the cedar abides even though the tree may be cut down and sawn into boards or beams or pillars. Hardly any wood unites so many good qualities as the cedar; its wood not only pleases the eye by its reddish stripes, and exhales an agreeable smell, but it is hard and without knots, and is never eaten by worms, and lasts so long that some persons consider it imperishable. Hence, in the typology of Scripture bespeaks the fragrance of His life – an eternal and incorruptible life!"

Spiritually, Cedar is symbolic of strength and serves as a hedge of protection. In Song of Solomon 1:17, it speaks about the boards of Cedarwood: *The beams of our house are cedar and our rafters of fir."* A bride's trousseau or "cedar chest," which holds her treasures, protects her valuables from moths, silverfish, and other infestations. A believer's heart is where God's treasure is. Yeshua reminds believers to guard their hearts against the enemy, who wants to come in and steal their joy and peace.

BIBLICAL REFERENCES TO CEDARWOOD

Leviticus 14:4
Leviticus 14:6
Leviticus 14:49
Leviticus 14:52
Numbers 19:6

CEDARWOOD (LUMBER)

2 Samuel 7:2
2 Samuel 7:7
1 Kings 5:8
1 Kings 6:9
1 Kings 6:10
1 Kings 6:15
1 Kings 6:16
1 Kings 6:18
1 Kings 6:20
1 Kings 6:36
1 Kings 7:2
1 Kings 7:3
1 Kings 7:7
1 Kings 7:12
1 Chronicles 14:1
1 Chronicles 17:1
1 Chronicles 17:6
1 Chronicles 22:4

2 Chronicles 2:3
Song of Solomon 1:17
Song of Solomon 8:9
Jeremiah 22:14
Jeremiah 22:15
Ezekiel 27:24
Zephaniah 2:14

CEDARWOOD (TREES)

Numbers 24:6
Judges 9:15
2 Samuel 5:11
1 Kings 4:33
1 Kings 5:6
1 Kings 5:10
1 Kings 7:11
1 Kings 9:11
1 Kings 10:27
2 Kings 14:9
2 Kings 19:23
1 Chronicles 22:4
2 Chronicles 1:15
2 Chronicles 2:8
2 Chronicles 9:27
2 Chronicles 25:18
Ezra 3:7
Job 40:17
Psalm 29:5
Psalm 80:20
Psalm 92:12

Psalm 104:16
Psalm 148:9
Song of Solomon 5:15
Isaiah 2:15
Isaiah 9:20
Isaiah 14:8
Isaiah 37:24
Isaiah 44:14
Jeremiah 22:7
Ezekiel 17:3
Ezekiel 17:22
Ezekiel 17:23
Ezekiel 31:3
Ezekiel 31:8
Amos 2:9
Zechariah 11:1
Zechariah 11:2

CEDARWOOD'S HEALING PROPERTIES

Cedrus Libani possesses an enormous trunk that can reach the height of 120 feet with a diameter of 9 feet. Such a massive trunk is often branching with a dense crown of dark green at the top, a characteristic in adult trees. Secondary branches are often ramified like a menorah.

According to an article entitled, "Cedars of Lebanon, Cedars of the Lord" on Habeeb.com's website, the Cedarwood tree is the most renowned natural monument in the universe. The writer describes how religion, poetry, and history all celebrate them. He states:

"The Arabs entertain a traditional veneration for these trees, attributing to them a vegetative power which enables them to live eternally, and an 'intelligence' which causes them to manifest signs of wisdom and foresight. They are said to understand the changes of the seasons as they stir their vast branches, inclining them towards heaven or earth accordingly as the snow proposes to fall or melt."

It is said that the snows have no sooner begun to fall than these Cedars turn their branches to rise insensibly, gathering their points upwards, forming, as it were, a pyramid or parasol. Assuming this new shape, they can sustain the immense weight of snow remaining upon them for so long.

The Egyptians used its resin to mummify their dead and thus called it the "life of death." Cedar sawdust was found in the tombs of the Pharaohs as well. Pharaohs and Pagans had the tradition of burning the cedar coming from Lebanon with their offerings and in their ceremonies. Jewish priests, however, were ordered by Moses to use the peel of the Lebanese Cedar in circumcision and for the treatment of leprosy. According to the Talmud, Jews used to burn Lebanese Cedarwood on the mountain of Olives announcing the beginning of the New Year.

Cedarwood has been used for over 5,000 years by ancient cultures such as the Egyptians and the Sumerians for ritual purposes. Other uses included embalming, a disinfectant, and other medicinal purposes. The superb qualities of the Cedarwood for its hardness, exquisite fragrance, bug resistance, and endurance to humidity and temperature encouraged the Phoenicians, Egyptians and Greeks and many others to use it extensively. It was the choice wood by the Phoenicians who built their trade ship and military fleets from Cedarwood, as well as the roofs of their temples and houses. Kings such as David and Solomon used it to build the Temple of Jerusalem and their Palaces. Cedarwood was also utilized in the temples and for furniture by the Assyrians and Babylonians. It is said that the Greeks and Romans had their share of Cedarwood, which they praised and had pride in.

TRADITIONAL USES

Cedarwood has been used for thousands of years in medicines and cosmetics. The Egyptians used it for embalming the dead. In Tibet, Cedarwood has been used for medicine and incense. The Scriptures record that Solomon built the Temple and his palace out of the Cedars of Lebanon – which may be why Solomon was the wisest man ever to live.

Cedarwood is emotionally calming and is known for its purifying properties. Cedarwood may be useful for anxiety, arthritis, congestion, coughs, cystitis, dandruff, psoriasis, hair loss, sinusitis, fluid retention, arteriosclerosis, ADHD, skin conditions such as acne, and other diseases.

For practical purposes, this oil serves well as an insect repellent. Its scent stays in the wood for a lifetime, even after the wood has been made into furniture – and it is this same fragrance that inhibits the growth of bacteria.

MEDICINAL USES

According to Valerie Gennari Cooksley at R.N. Aromatherapy, Cedarwood is effective against hair loss, tuberculosis, bronchitis, gonorrhea, urinary infections, acne, and psoriasis. A study conducted by America Academy of Reflexology showed it also helps in reducing the hardening of the artery wall.

Cedarwood stimulates the limbic region of the brain (the center of emotions) and the pineal gland, which releases melatonin for deep sleep. Terry Friedmann, M.D. found in clinical tests that this oil was able to successfully treat ADD and ADHD (attention deficit disorders) in children. It is recognized for its calming, purifying properties.

In reflexology, the thumb and big toe are trigger points for clearing fears of the unknown and mental blocks against learning. The big toe is also a point for clearing addictions and compulsive behavior. The scent of Cedarwood helps to clear buried emotions, including pride and conceit.

Cedarwood contains 98% sesquiterpenes, which oxygenates the brain and deletes or erases misinformation written in the DNA as a result of trauma, abuse, loss, ancestral or generational behaviors, and limiting beliefs. Sesquiterpenes are considered the antidepressant in this valuable aspect. Cedarwood may also be useful as a general cerebral stimulant.

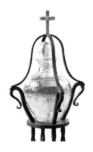

Cinnamon

Cinnamon appears in four places in the Bible and also extensively in Rabbinic writings. True Cinnamon comes from a tree belonging to the Lauraceae family and has long, oval green leaves. It bears fruit, which grows on stalks and looks like tiny black cherries. The Cinnamon used for culinary and medicinal purposes is taken from the inner bark of the tree.

The old Latin name was *Cinnamonum zeolanicum* named after Sri Lanka's former name Ceylon. To this day, Sri Lanka still produces between 80-90% of the world's Cinnamon harvest, although it is also cultivated in Madagascar and the Seychelles.

What is important to note here is that it is a long way from Israel.

The first time Cinnamon is mentioned in the Scriptures is when Moses is instructed to make an anointing oil for the priest's garments and the furnishings of the Tabernacle. In Exodus 32:22-24 its says,

> *Moreover, the LORD spoke to Moses, saying, Take also for yourself the finest of spices: of flowing Myrrh five hundred shekels, and of fragrant Cinnamon half as much, two hundred and fifty, and of fragrant cane two hundred and fifty, and of Cassia five hundred, according to the shekel of the sanctuary, and of Olive oil a hin.*

The finest of spices: perhaps those with the most pungent scent? You will note God mentions not only Cinnamon but also Cassia. Cinnamon and its cheaper counterpart, Cassia, are often confused and yet here God is clear – Cinnamon is finer, and so he requires only half as much.

The question is, though, how did the Israelites get hold of this ingredient when it grew so far away? We know there were spice merchants along the Incense Trail, but for this recipe to work, this would have to have been oil. Perhaps it was traded in Egypt, or the Israelites had learned the perfumery process. What is known is that the Egyptians by this period were already master perfumers. Every Egyptian home would have housed some Cinnamon, as it was so widely used as medicine.

The Lord instructed, *You shall speak to the sons of Israel, saying, 'This shall be a holy anointing oil to Me throughout your generations.*

So he expects there will be an endless supply of Cinnamon to treat the generations to come; nevertheless, the edict is clear. This is a holy oil and should not be used for any other common purpose.

This has two meanings for Israelites. The first is certain. This oil sets you apart as chosen people. This Cinnamon, along with other spices, is an ingredient considered worthy as a worshipful tool for Yahweh. This choice sets the Israelites apart.

Later in 1 Samuel 8:13 there is a clear warning about lavish living for the Israelites. He warns about the rulership of kings, but many commentators suggest the word *Pharaohs* works better here:

> *He will appoint for himself commanders of thousands and of fifties, and some to do his plowing and to reap his harvest and to make his weapons of war and equipment for his chariots. He will also take your daughters for perfumers and cooks and bakers. He will take the best of your fields and your vineyards and your Olive groves and give them to his servants.*

Does the verse also warn of the dangers of lavish living taking away the reverence of Yahweh? After all, an Israelite could have but one ruler, his God.

Our next encounter with the spicy scent of Cinnamon is in Solomon's enchanting love song. In Song of Solomon 7:13-15, it reads,

> Your shoots are an orchard of pomegranates with choice fruits, henna with nard plants, Nard, and Saffron, Calamus and Cinnamon, with all the trees of Frankincense, Myrrh, and Aloes, along with all the finest spices. You are a garden spring, a well of fresh water, and streams flowing from Lebanon.

In other translations, the word *orchard* is replaced by *locked garden*, which takes on a whole different exotic tone. A secret pleasure, a preciously guarded taboo, rich and juicy – and, of course, we also have the modern meaning of a very spicy tale.

But there was another orchard, another garden locked preciously away, wasn't there? Some commentators suggest this has an alignment with Eden itself – a blissful retreat back to God.

Around A.D. 200, there was written a set of Jewish pseudepigraphical texts. These included the Apocalypse of Moses and the Life of Adam and Eve. In the Apocalypse, Adam pleads with the angels to let him "return to Paradise to take herbs as an offering to God that he might hear me." The list of plants allowed included Crocus (obviously the source of saffron), Nard, Calamus, and Cinnamon – the same list as we see in the Song of Solomon.

Later in the Life of Adam and Eve, Eve and Seth plead again, this time to the Archangel Michael for these same herbs for an anointing oil.

In fact, it is cited so many times in Rabbinic texts as having been one of the trees of Paradise, after the Bar Khobar revolt in the First Jewish War (132-136 B.C.) they began to talk of the land where "goats feed on the Cinnamon tree" as a reference to their own homeland.

This tone of sheer delightfulness of Cinnamon is continued in Proverbs 4:14 but had an entirely more wanton element to it. The adulterous woman proclaims of her former life in Proverbs 4:6-18,

> I have spread my couch with coverings, with colored linens of Egypt. I have sprinkled my bed with Myrrh, Aloes, and Cinnamon. Come, let us drink our fill of love until morning; Let us delight ourselves with caresses.

In the book of Proverbs, it gives a hint to its meaning. Proverbs 7:17 says, *I have perfumed my bed with Myrrh, Aloes, and Cinnamon.*

The primary root of the word Cinnamon means "emitting an odor," while spiritually in the Bible it speaks of holiness and set-apartness. In the Song of Solomon, Cinnamon grows in a locked garden that Yeshua calls "my sister, my bride" in Song of Solomon 4:12-14.

For every new believer, the heart is a fragrant garden, enclosed and set apart for him alone. We must allow the Father to form and shape us into the image of him and share the heart of the Lord that is undivided in devotion to him. 2 Corinthians 2:14-15 says,

> *Thanks be to God, who always leads us in triumph in Christ, and manifests through us the sweet aroma of the knowledge of Him in every place. For we are a fragrance of Christ to God.*

It is not clear if oil or powder was used here, but Cinnamon on the bed is more than purely fragrant, it would heighten sensitivity in the most eye-watering of ways! One commentator Robert Connell suggests there is a grizzlier connotation not immediately evident to modern eyes. He wonders at how much burial practices have changed over the centuries. The Bible is rife with tales of bodies being wrapped in shrouds of spiced sheets, not the least Christ himself. Was the promiscuous foreign woman using Cinnamon to lure her lover to a blissful petite mort or a more literal sense of death itself?

We do not hear of the spice again until its fragrance pervades the New Testament in Revelation 18:12-14. Here the writer creates a thinly veiled barb, using the name Babylon, but very clearly pointing his finger at Rome:

> *...cargoes of gold and silver and precious stones and pearls and fine linen and purple and silk and scarlet, and every*

kind of citron wood and every article of ivory and every article made from very costly wood and bronze and iron and marble, and Cinnamon and spice and incense and perfume and Frankincense and wine and Olive oil and fine flour and wheat and cattle and sheep, and cargoes of horses and chariots and slaves and human lives. The fruit you long for has gone from you, and all things that were luxurious and splendid have passed away from you and men will no longer find them.

This righteous indignation is fueled by his fervent belief that Rome has pillaged the land of his ancestors, that botanical wealth and human labor should not belong to Rome, and that merchants have benefitted from this disgrace. The wealth correctly belongs to the New Jerusalem and decrees Babylon/Rome will pay with judgment of the New Kingdom of Christ.

Works by Pliny contemporaneous to the book of Revelation show Cinnamon to be at the very top of their indulgent love for luxuries. The lowly spice spread across the globe and no wonder it was so revered. To have been desired on the opposite side of the planet from its source, thousands of years before anyone would recognize the name of Ceylon and to be the very ingredient required to communicate with God. A fascinating spice history indeed.

BIBLICAL REFERENCES TO CINNAMON

Exodus 30:23
Proverbs 7:17
Song of Solomon 4:14

CINNAMON'S HEALING PROPERTIES

Cinnamomum zeylanicum, Cinnamon's botanical name, comes from trees native to China and South East Asia. Its use is recorded in Chinese journals as early as 2700 B.C. During the middle ages, the Arabs that traded Cinnamon preserved their spice trade monopoly by claiming it was harvested from the nest of ferocious birds. Many believe Cinnamon attracts wealth and prosperity.

Obtained from its bark or leaf, the reddish-brown spicy oil warms the heart with its ability to help the melancholia and lift one's spirit from depression caused by lethargy and lack of vitality.

Cinnamon Bark essential oil is revered for its antiseptic properties and its pleasant spicy scent. It is best known for the treatment of stomach ailments (gas, diarrhea, upset stomach). This oil has the ability to combat viral and infectious diseases. Research has been unable to find a virus, bacteria, or fungus that can live in the presence of Cinnamon.

In the book *Cinnamon and Cassia*, by P. N. Ravindran, K. Nirmal Babu, and M. Shylaja, they state:

"The different investigations reveal that Cinnamon shows both immune system potentiating and inhibiting effects…Kaishi-ni-eppi-ichi tu, (TJS-664) a Chinese herbal preparation containing Cinnamon as its principal constituent, has been shown to exhibit antiviral action against the influenza A2 virus."

The Journal of Agricultural and Food Chemistry has reported Cinnamon oil is an excellent mosquito repellent, because of its high concentration of cinnamaldehyde, an active mosquito-killing agent.

It also makes a great room freshener because of its strong aroma. Cinnamon blends well with Frankincense, Lavender and Onycha (Benzoin).

Because of its high phenol content, it is best diluted (1 drop to 40 or 50 drops of a quality oil, such as extra-virgin Olive oil) before applying on the skin. If the mixture is too hot, use additional diluting oil.

TRADITIONAL USES

This prized spice was used by a band of thieves who stole jewels off dead bodies during the Black Plague in Europe without contracting the disease. When the King of England questioned them, he discovered that their secret was essential oils, which included Cinnamon.

This spicy, warm oil is used for lifting of spirits and reducing glucose. Cinnamon is used extensively in cooking and flavoring of beverages.

MEDICINAL USES

Cinnamon is good for the digestive system, calms spasms, lower high blood pressure, eases colitis, flatulence, diarrhea, and nausea. It is known to ease muscular spasms and painful rheumatic joints, as well as general aches and pains. It also affects the libido and is known as an aphrodisiac. Several studies suggest that Cinnamon may have a regulatory effect on blood sugar, making it especially beneficial for people with type II diabetes. In some studies, Cinnamon has shown an amazing ability to stop medication-resistant yeast infections. In a study published by researchers at the U.S. Department of Agriculture in Maryland, Cinnamon reduced the proliferation of leukemia and lymphoma cancer cells. It has shown to have an anti-clotting effect on the blood.

Other properties include antimicrobial, anti-infectious, antibacterial (for broad spectrum of infection), antiseptic, anti-inflammatory, antiviral, antifungal, anticoagulant, antidepressant, and emotional stimulant. It is also used for fungal infections (Candida), as a general tonic, and it is known to increase blood flow where previously restricted.

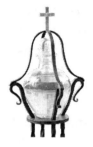

Coriander

Coriander, or Cilantro, is a member of the Apiaceae family. It is also sometimes known as Chinese Parsley and is native to Southern Europe, North Africa, and Southwest Asia. It has wispy fern-like leaves and tiny umbel flowers of either white or sometimes very pale pink.

The plant has two edible sources: the leaves, which have a fresh citrus flavor, and the seeds, which have a muskier lemony citrus taste. Strangely, many people do not taste the leaves as fresh; some experience a soap-like taste. This is a genetic trait of not being able to discern the taste of unsaturated aldehydes.

Coriander is mentioned twice in the Bible. On both occasions, it refers to the similarity of the seeds in their appearance to their manna from heaven. The first instance is in Exodus 16:31,

> *So the people rested on the seventh day. The house of Israel named it manna, and it was like coriander seed, white, and its taste was like wafers with honey. Then Moses said, This is what the LORD had commanded, Let an omerful of it be kept throughout your generations, that they may see the bread that I fed you in the wilderness when I brought you out of the land of Egypt.*

The second time is in Numbers 11:7,

> *...but now our appetite is gone. There is nothing at all to look at except this manna. Now the manna was like coriander seed and its appearance like that of bdellium. The people would go about and gather it and grind it between two millstones or beat it in the mortar, and boil it in the pot and make cakes with it, and its taste was as the taste of cakes baked with oil.*

There is a deeper meaning hidden according to scholars. The Hebrew word translated as Coriander actually means "to cut." The way Coriander grows furrowed in the soil reminded the Israelites of the way a cut heals in gathers. But this metaphor doesn't relate to just any cut, it relates to a self-inflicted wound.

In 1 Kings 18, Elijah was challenged by 450 prophets of Baal to see whose god was real. They challenged him to call fire down from heaven to light up a sacrifice of a bull. Leading the way, the prophets of Baal prayed and wailed and danced around, but their God did not show. Then in verse 28 it says,

> *And they cried aloud, and cut themselves*
> *after their manner with knives and lancets,*
> *till the blood gushed out upon them.*

Zealous cutting was very much a part of the devotional worship of the time. The humble would request of God to look favorably on their self-mutilation. You will note another Jewish cut, that of circumcision: cutting the foreskin to symbolize cutting sin from their lives.

In modern day Judaism, Coriander is still used as one of the bitter herbs of Passover.

Archeologists have found evidence of Coriander way back to the early Neolithic period where 15 desiccated mericarps were found in the Nahal Hemel Cave in Israel. They had also been found in many other archeological discoveries in Egypt, most notably in the pyramids and a ½ liter of mericarps was found in the tomb of Tutankhamen. Clearly this was an herb they felt would be of use in the afterlife. Coriander, however, was not native to Egypt, and so we know even in those early days it was being cultivated in the land of the Pharaohs.

One of the main reasons for this cultivation, apart from its digestive prowess in culinary and medicinal uses, was perhaps its importance in the manufacture of perfumery. The Linear B tablets of Pylos show how highly it was revered in fragrance throughout Greece as early as the 2nd Millennium B.C. Indeed later in his writings, Pliny described the very best Coriander coming from Egypt.

Coriander was well loved by the Romans as well. They brought it from Europe with them to preserve their meats and would use it extensively to flavor their bread. The Chinese linked the herb with immortality, and in the Middle Ages, Coriander was used across Europe to flavor love potions.

BIBLICAL REFERENCES TO CORIANDER

Exodus 16:31
Numbers 11:7

CORIANDER'S HEALING PROPERTIES

Coriander is a favorite herb, widely used as a garnish and flavoring in cookery. It is thought to be one of the oldest herbs in the world and has been popular throughout history as a medicinal remedy. Coriander seeds were also discovered in Egyptian tombs and are mentioned in the Bible as a comparison to manna. Traditionally, it was also one of the bitter *maror* herbs eaten at the Passover.

Today, Coriander continues to be an essential ingredient for fragrance and flavor in a range of pharmaceutical products, toiletries, and perfumes. In domestic cookery, Coriander (or Cilantro) is a favorite ingredient in curries, salads, and Mexican dishes.

Coriander is native to Europe and western Asia, particularly around the Holy Land region. Like many other herbs and aromatic plants, Coriander belongs to the Apiaceae family. The essential oil is steam distilled from the seeds of the plant and has a sweet, spicy scent. As a middle note, Coriander is a versatile oil for blending in aromatherapy and combines well with Clary Sage, Bergamot, Jasmine, Neroli, Sandalwood, Cypress, Pine and other spice oils.

TRADITIONAL USES

Coriander was often used as a remedy for indigestion. It was thought to boost fertility and was often placed on women's legs during labor to ease childbirth. As an aphrodisiac, Coriander was also used in medieval love potions.

MEDICINAL USES

Coriander is most commonly used to treat digestive disorders, such as diarrhea, flatulence, nausea, loss of appetite and indigestion. As a stimulant, it boosts the circulation, which helps to eliminate fluid retention and accumulated toxins. The analgesic nature of Coriander makes it a useful oil for treating muscular aches and pains, migraines and neuralgia. Emotionally, Coriander can boost poor memory and help to tackle stress and low confidence.

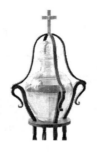

Cumin

Cumin is a member of the parsley family, closely related to the Cow Parsley and Queen Anne's lace we see growing wild in the hedgerows. It is an annual plant that grows to around 30 centimeters tall. The seeds we eat are actually the fruit of the plant.

Throughout history, it has been known by very similar names. The Hebrews called it *kamon*, and in Arabic, it is referred to as *kemum*. Its name comes from the Greek word *kyminom*.

Cumin appears three times in the Bible. Two occurrences are very close together in Isaiah and then it is mentioned again in the New Testament. In Isaiah 28:27 it says,

When he has leveled the surface, does he not sow caraway and scatter cumin? Does he not plant wheat in its place, barley in its plot, and spelt in its field?

For the fitches are not threshed with a threshing instrument, neither is a cart wheel turned about upon the cumin; but the fitches are beaten out with a staff, and the cumin with a rod.

Here Isaiah passionately speaks about faith in the Lord at times when he tests us. He explains adversity comes in many guises because different situations require different measures. Cumin seeds are laden with volatile oils and so harvesting them is a very delicate operation. The Cumin is a metaphor for how hard a lesson is as a measure of our strength. Sometimes a slight nudge might be enough, sometimes he threatens, corrects, and, of course, shows mercy.

It is important to remember the Old Testament Lord is described as very different from who we know today. The Israelites knew him to be vengeful, omnipotent and sometimes even cruel. It was because of him they endured fire, floods, pestilence and plague. Only with the dawn of Christ's New Kingdom was there any sentiment of forgiveness.

But why must we learn these lessons? Isaiah explains these are his way of separating us away from the crowd. When we ask for help, we grow closer to him. We also look inside of ourselves and discover things we did not know. He is preparing us for use. At the end of days, he will gather up his harvest, and the chaff will be burned in the unquenchable fire.

There is also a reference to "fitches." This is believed to pertain to the so-called *Black Cumin Nigella Sativum*, a sweeter version of Cumin, also known as the Black Onion Seed.

In the New Testament Cumin is mentioned in the verse describing how Jesus decries the Pharisees in the temple. Matthew 23:23 says,

> *Woe to you, teachers of the law and Pharisees, you hypocrites! You give a tenth of your spices - mint, dill, and cumin. But you have neglected the more important matters of the law - justice, mercy, and faithfulness. You should have practiced the latter, without neglecting the former.*

Cumin was not only a well-loved seasoning, but it was also a currency of tithing to the temple. It is known Cumin grew well in Israel but was inferior in quality to that grown in Ethiopia (Pliny). However, it was in plentiful supply. It was then such a simple tithe to pay; meaningless almost, in Jesus' eyes. Rather than being consumed by love for the Lord, they paid their dues in seeds.

The symbolism of Cumin at the time is relevant here, too. Egyptian women wore Cumin as a hope of conception from intercourse. Sailors, soldiers, and indeed spice merchants would carry Cumin seeds in their pockets as a remembrance of faithfulness of those whom they had left behind. Faithful, but not passionate, not engulfed by the fire of love; no wonder the Pharisees had Jesus riled.

HISTORICAL FINDS OF CUMIN

Archaeological finds in India found seeds dating back to the 2nd millennium B.C. In Egypt, it has been found at sites dating as far back as the New Kingdom (16-11,000 B.C.). Both Nigella and Cumin seeds were found in Tutankhamen's tomb, leading some sources to suggest both may have been used in the embalming process.

The Romans and Greeks used Cumin extensively in their cooking, not least because it was a far cheaper alternative to pepper. The ancient Greeks would keep a table condiment of Cumin much like we do with pepper today. This tradition continues in some parts of Morocco.

Because it was cheaper, in Rome Cumin came to be synonymous with frugality and economizing, especially in connection with the greedy obsession of gaining wealth. The emperor Antonius Pius gained the nickname Cumin Seed "Splitter" because of his austerity measures. Some attribute the name Marcus Cuminus to his successor Marcus Aurelius, perhaps not because of his greed (since this does not go well with his posthumous title, the Philosopher) but more for his dislike of wasteful living.

An interesting quote is derived from the Quran when the Prophet Mohammed, peace be upon him, says, "Use the Black Seed for indeed, it is a cure for every disease except death" (Saheeh al-Bukharee 7:591).

BIBLICAL REFERENCES TO CUMIN

Isaiah 28:25
Isaiah 28:27a
Isaiah 28:27b
Matthew 23:23

CUMIN'S HEALING PROPERTIES

Cumin seeds have been spread far and wide across the globe for many a millennia. There are two pools of thought about where their native home might have been. One school says Turkestan; another, the Upper Nile lands.

The warming scent of Cumin is familiar as a culinary spice and key ingredient in curry dishes. Native to Egypt and the Mediterranean region, Cumin is part of the Apiaceae family, along with its close relation Coriander.

The essential oil is produced from the seeds of the plant through a process of steam distillation. The warm, spicy scent acts as a middle-base note that blends well with other spice oils, as well as Lavender, Rosemary, and Rosewood.

TRADITIONAL USES

Its use dates back to ancient times, with evidence of Cumin seeds found at Egyptian archeological sites. Cumin was – and still is – traditionally used as a digestive aid in Ayurvedic medicine. The spice is mentioned in the Bible, as the Pharisees paid their taxes with tithes of Cumin. It was also used as a currency during the Middle Ages before it became widely available as a domestic spice.

MEDICINAL USES

While Cumin is most notable for its use as a digestive aid, it is also beneficial for treating muscular problems and nervous disorders. Massaging the diluted essential oil can help to relieve headaches, arthritis, and muscular pains. Its stimulant properties can help to boost the circulation, improving blood flow and encouraging the elimination of toxins and excess fluid. As a nervine oil, Cumin can be useful for strengthening the nervous system and helping with debility and nervous exhaustion.

SPICE CHEST: TITHES

Many of the herbs cited in this book result from two passages in the New Testament where Jesus accuses the Pharisees of being careful in their tithes of herbs, but not asserting themselves passionately enough in their love of God.

But what is this tithe?

The Hebrew word for *tithe* means ten percent and the Hebrews were compelled by Mosaic Law to give a tithe to the temple in reverence to God. It is, however, a misconception their commitment was for a mere 10%. Just as today we are obliged to pay several taxes, so were the Israelites.

In Numbers 18:20 we learn the first tithe of the year is specifically to go to the Levitical priesthood, and this is listed as a 10th of one's earnings.

In Deuteronomy 12:1-19 and 14:22-26, we read of a second yearly tithe, which came at the time of the feasts. The Israelites are instructed to take the first born of their flocks and herd and also a portion of their grain, new wines, and oils.

But in Deuteronomy 14:28, a three-year tithe to the poor is also expected. Calculating this at a third of ten percent and because it happened once every three years, we can now see the tithe for an Israelite amounted to 23.3% per year.

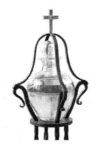

Cypress

Cupressus sempervirens is commonly referred to as Cypress essential oil of the Cupressaceae family and is also called Italian or Mediterranean Cypress.

The tree is an evergreen tree, conical-shaped, about 28 meters (80 feet) high. Originating from the East, it's now mostly found in gardens and cemeteries in the Mediterranean region. It has dark green foliage, small flowers and round brown-grey cones with seed nuts inside. The wood is hard and durable, red-yellow in color.

The Phoenicians and Cretans used the wood for building ships and houses while the Egyptians made sarcophagi from it and the Greeks used it to carve statues of their gods. In fact, Cypress was devoted to Pluto, Roman God of the Underworld.

The Greek word *Sempervirens*, from which the botanical name is derived, means "lives forever" and the tree also gave its name to the island of Cypress, where it used to be worshiped.

It is believed that the cross of Jesus had been made of Cypress wood, as the tree generally seems to be associated with death.

Just as Cedarwood is symbolic of strength, Cypress is also known for strength and durability. These trees were described in the apocryphal book of Sirach as "trees which groweth up to the clouds." The Hebrew word for "Cypress" is *tirzah*, which means "make slender."

The Bible tells that the wood used for Noah's ark was "gopher wood or cypress" in Genesis 6:14:

> *Make thee an ark of gopher wood; rooms*
> *shalt thou make in the ark, and shalt pitch*
> *it within and without with pitch.*

It is believed to be Cypress because of its ability to stand up to adverse conditions. Building anything that big would require trees that reached the clouds!

Isaiah 60:13 tells how Cypress represents the sanctuary of the holy feet of God in the coming messianic kingdom: *The glory of Lebanon shall come unto thee, the fir tree, the pine tree, and the box together, to beautify the place of my sanctuary; and I will make the place of my feet glorious.*

BIBLICAL REFERENCES TO CYPRESS

Genesis 6:14
Isaiah 41:19
Isaiah 44:14
1 Kings 9:11
Song of Solomon 1:17

CYPRESS' HEALING PROPERTIES

Cypress has been used since ancient times for purification and as incense. Cypress essential oil is one of the oils most used for the circulatory system because it assists in moving stagnant matter. It actually assists many systems of the body including the circulatory, digestive, urinary, and integumentary (skin). It helps with cellulite, varicose veins, hemorrhoids, fluid retention, constipation, edema, excessive perspiration, and hand and feet sweating. Cypress is also effective for muscles and joints, the respiratory system, the reproductive system, and the nervous system.

TRADITIONAL USES

Cypress is one of the oils most used for the circulatory system. The therapeutic qualities of Cypress include improving circulation, supporting the nerves and intestines, and supporting the immune system and cardiovascular system. Cypress essential oil was used for centuries to alleviate menstrual problems because of its ability to circulate and regulate blood flow.

MEDICINAL USES

Cypress is a good defense against arthritis, bronchitis, cramps, hemorrhoids, insomnia, intestinal parasites, menopausal symptoms, menstrual pain, pancreas inefficiencies, pulmonary infections, throat problems, varicose veins, fluid retention, and scar tissue. It is known to be anti-infectious, antibacterial, and antimicrobial. It strengthens blood capillaries and is good for teeth and gums.

This oil considered anti-infectious, antibacterial, antimicrobial, and strengthens blood capillaries. It also acts as an insect repellent.

Jean Valnet, M.D. suggests that it may be helpful for some cancers. This oil may be beneficial for improving energy, reducing cellulite, strengthening connective tissue, asthma, coughs, edema, gallbladder, bleeding gums, hemorrhaging, laryngitis, liver disorders, muscular cramps, nervous tension, nose bleeds, and ovarian cysts. It is outstanding when used in skin care, lessening scar tissue.

Cypress' ORAC value is 24,300 µTE/100g. (ORAC stands for Oxygen Radical Absorbance Capacity and tells you the antioxidant capacity of a food item. Antioxidants have shown to reduce the risk of age-related conditions and cancer.)

Cypress helps ease the feeling of loss and creates a sense of security. It also brings healing to one during emotional trauma.

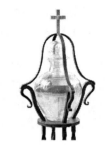

Dill

There is debate whether Dill is mentioned in the Bible. In Matthew 23:23, Jesus may have referred to Dill or alternatively another translation might be Anise, *Pimpella anisum*. Today, it is mostly held the plant cited was Dill.

Dill is an annual plant of the celery family. It belongs to the family Apiaceae and is the only plant in the genus Anethum. It is a willowy plant with hollow slender stems topped with soft, delicate leaves. It grows to a height of around 30-40 centimeters tall.

As we have seen many times throughout this book, in the verse in Matthew Jesus challenges the Pharisees' commitment to God by their dedication to tithing seeds to the temple over fervent acts of love.

Dill was a well-used plant in biblical times for exactly the same reasons we use it today, its ability to relieve wind. The herb used in babies' gripe water is described at length in the Ebers Papyrus, found in 1810, dating back to 1500 B.C. It translates from hieroglyphs as "soothes flatulence, relieves dyspepsia, laxative and diuretic properties."

When the tomb of the great Amenhotep II was opened, there were stalks of Dill, which had been entombed there with him since his ritual burial in 1401 B.C.

We know Dill originated from Russia and had been used for its medicinal purposes for over 5,000 years. Since this time it has been used as an aphrodisiac and in the Middle Ages, it was hung over babies' cots to ward off witches!

The ancient Greeks used Dill as their symbol of wealth, and the Romans believed it to be a bringer of good fortune, weaving it into the wreaths of their athletes.

Today most of us know Dill either for Gripe Water or Dill Pickles. For this, we have King Charles I of England to thank. In 1640, he requested Dill be added to his pickled cucumbers!

BIBLICAL REFERENCES TO DILL

Isaiah 28:25
Isaiah 28:27
Matthew 23:23

DILL'S HEALING PROPERTIES

As a popular medicinal and culinary herb since ancient times, Dill is most commonly known for being a digestive aid. Native to the Mediterranean and the Black Sea region, the aromatic herb belongs to the Apiaceae botanical family.

Dill essential oil is extracted from the seeds of the plant by steam distillation. Its chemical composition varies between chemotypes, but the principal constituent is usually carvone. The aroma of Dill is fresh, sweet, spicy and slightly grassy. It is classed as a middle note in aromatherapy and blends well with spice oils, as well as Elemi, Mint, Caraway, Nutmeg, and Bergamot.

The soothing property of Dill was recognized by the Anglo-Saxons, who named the herb *dylle*, which means "to lull." Previously, it was a traditional herbal remedy for the ancient Egyptians, Greeks and Romans. In biblical times, Dill was used as a form of currency. Today, Dill continues to be a favorite ingredient in German and Scandinavian cuisine.

TRADITIONAL USES

Not only is Dill a biblical herb, but its use stems back to ancient civilizations. The earliest evidence of its medicinal use dates back to Egyptian manuscripts written 5,000 years ago.

The Greeks made perfume from Dill leaves, and athletes massaged the oil over their bodies as a muscle tonic. In ancient Rome, gladiators used Dill to calm their nerves before battles.

During the medieval period, Dill was hung over doorframes to ward off witchcraft and tied to bedposts to aid insomnia. Herbalists traditionally prescribed Dill for jaundice, headaches, boils, nausea, liver problems and stomach complaints. It was a popular digestive remedy for babies and children when prepared as "Dill water," similar to gripe water.

MEDICINAL USES

Dill is predominantly used to treat digestive complaints, such as constipation, bloating, cramps, and heartburn. It may help to regulate blood sugar levels stated by the *Complete Herbal Guide: A Natural Approach to Healing the Body*. Dill also has antibacterial properties that help to fight intestinal micro-organisms such as Staphylococcus aureus.

Dill can also be a useful remedy against hiccups as it soothes the diaphragm contractions that cause the condition. This soothing, antispasmodic quality also helps with menstrual cramps, high blood pressure, and general tension. The relaxing aroma of Dill has the ability to calm the mind, and may even have an aphrodisiac effect.

The estrogen-like effects of Dill can help to stimulate menstruation and encourage lactation.

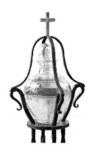

Fennel

Fennel is yet another suggestion as to the herb
sometimes described as "fitches" in Isaiah 28:25. Its soft,
feathery leaves might also have perhaps been Caraway
or Dill. Here Isaiah discusses God's dealings with his
people and how they will come to follow and trust in his
word instinctively. He describes how the farmer already
intuitively understands the laws of nature; that God's
instruction can always be relied upon to show the way.
In Isaiah 28:25 he asks,

> *Fennel isn't threshed with a threshing-*
> *sledge, nor is a cart wheel rolled over*
> *cumin, but fennel is beaten with a staff,*
> *and cumin with a rod.*

Despite its virtual invisibility in the Bible, Fennel was a vital part of Jewish cuisine. This is made apparent to the references in several ancient Hebrew texts. The leaves were used as a spice similar manner to Dill. Fennel is called *gufnan* in the Mishnah (Dem. 1:1) and *shumar* in the Talmud. The Jerusalem Talmud (Dem. 1:1, 21d) describes how Galileans did not consider it a spice, but that it was regarded as such in Judah.

The word *kezah* does appear in the Bible and other contemporaneous literature, and although not officially ascribed, it has been suggested it may have been the seed of the Fennel flower. It is thought that it was used as a spice on bread.

BIBLICAL REFERENCES TO FENNEL

Isaiah 28:25

FENNEL'S HEALING PROPERTIES

Fennel essential oil is extracted from the seeds of the plant by steam distillation. Its name comes from the Greek, meaning "hay," and it grows to almost 2 meters in height.

The vegetable is rich in vitamin C. A cupful will provide 20% of the daily nutritional requirement. It also provides a rich source of potassium, which acts a vasodilator in the body. This relaxes the walls of the blood vessels reducing constriction on blood pressure and circulatory problems such as varicose veins.

The seeds contain an amino acid called histidine, which stimulates the body to make hemoglobin, meaning Fennel is the aromatic medicine of choice for people suffering from anemia. There is growing evidence that the seeds may have chemo-protective properties.

TRADITIONAL USES

Throughout the Mediterranean, people chew Fennel seeds to freshen their breath after eating and to aid digestion. The seed extract is universally used in toothpaste.

Medieval herbals all seem to agree that medicinal usage appears to have originally come from Italy. There it is, even today, used and sliced very thinly into salads to aid digestion. Although it is found in some Roman cookbooks, it does not seem as if it was cultivated in Northern Europe at the time. The Chinese and Egyptians both held it in very high regard believing it would ward off evil spirits.

There are many Anglo-Saxon references to it being used in England, which predate the Normal conquest in A.D. 1066. It seems the poorest people would add it to their food to make it more palatable during Lent and would supplement it to make meals go further when food was sparse.

MEDICINAL USES

Fennel balances hormonal problems and is used to regulate periods. It has a strong diuretic action, which is excellent from releasing water retention but also swellings and edema throughout the body.

Its digestive properties are superlative. Fennel relieves flatulence, indigestion, and constipation as well as colic and diarrhea.

It is a wonderful respiratory tonic, alleviating restriction in the bronchial tracts, and also expelling catarrh and phlegm build-up.

A decoction of Fennel is used as a cooling lotion for puffy eyes, aiding their detoxification and lymphatic drainage.

Emotionally it is an extremely fortifying oil. It sustains courage and convictions and helps a person stand firm in adversity.

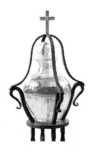

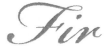

The Fir of the Bible is the Hebrew word *berosh*. Often it is translated as Fir, but most commentators suggest it is better listed as Cypress or even Cedar. There are clues throughout the Old Testament that fit like a jigsaw puzzle to lead us to this conclusion.

The controversy begins with Isaiah 60:30 when the passage names the Fir tree in a list alongside the Cypress. Here commentators suggest it should be better attributed to the Cedar, a tree growing well right across the Lebanon, and here we have an exact location given. In Isaiah 60:30 NIV it reads,

The glory of Lebanon will come to you, the juniper, the fir and the cypress together, to adorn my sanctuary; and I will glorify the place for my feet.

In the famous Jewish sermon by Charles Haddon Spurgeon at the Metropolitan Synagogue in 1864, he speaks of how God compares himself to a Fir tree in this verse: *From me is thy fruit found.* The grand Fir spreads its magnificent branches and provides shade and shelter from the burning sun. But man cannot live there for long because the Fir does not provide food and the shelter would not last forever. For this eternal sustenance, man must turn to God.

What is known from the passage in Isaiah 41:19 is that it was considered a tree of practical use. The planting of the Fir improved the area.

In 2 Kings 19:23, again we hear of the love for the tree, but this time, the translator is clear this tree, *berosh*, is the Cypress.

The fact that Fir tree crops were ravaged for sales to Egypt in order for them to build temples to their profane gods is seen as an insult to the Lord. So why might this be? Later we read in 1 Kings 6:15 this wood is an excellent construction tool – it is long, wide and extremely straight, so much so, floors were made of it:

The entire inside, from floor to ceiling, was paneled with wood. He paneled the walls and ceilings with cedar, and he used planks of cypress for the floors.

The ceiling of the temple, the highest point the Israelites could reach toward God, was covered with *behosh*. This marked the point where they were physically closest to God.

We know from papyri during this time in Egypt, their tallest native tree was the Acacia, which was not tall enough for the dictates of an Egyptian building. Their regulations required planks to be at least 4 meters long for rafters and shipbuilding. Therefore, they needed to import large amounts of wood from the Lebanon. Can you imagine the Israelites disgust? Their precious *berosh* sold for the glory of the Egyptian gods of profanity? The wood was a treasured product, and now the Egyptians were prepared to pay good money for it. Their money must have been impossible to resist, despite the sour taste it left in their mouths. No wonder the Israelites saw its trade as distasteful.

In Ezekiel 31:8, the Fir tree is used a metaphor for the corruption of Egypt and the prediction of its fall:

> *So it was beautiful in its greatness, in the length of its branches; for its roots extended to many waters. The cedars in God's garden could not match it; the cypresses could not compare with its boughs, and the plane trees could not match its branches. No tree in God's garden could compare with it in its beauty. I made it beautiful with the multitude of its branches, and all the trees of Eden, which were in the garden of God, were jealous of it.*

Like many civilizations ruined through sinful behavior, the narrator expects the same will come to Egypt. She is compared with the most beautiful of trees, reaching far and wide. But she will not last.

In Ezekiel 6:5 we see Fir also listed as wood for instruments worthy of playing to the Lord, but there seems to be no other evidence this was common use:

> *Meanwhile, David and all the house of Israel were celebrating before the LORD with all kinds of instruments made of fir wood, and with lyres, harps, tambourines, castanets, and cymbals. But when they came to the threshing-floor of Nacon, Uzzah reached out toward the ark of God and took hold of it, for the oxen nearly upset it.*

So the tree *berosh* is sometimes ambiguous. Could it be the Fir tree we now know so well? Certainly the description could just as easily relate to *Pinus hapiensis*, the tree we attribute to Pine. They are, after all, very closely related. More likely, historians feel it could be one of two species of the Cupressineae family, one of which is the *Cupressus semperivens*, the aromatherapist's beloved Cypress.

Adding weight to this claim are archeological discoveries in Egypt of how they viewed Cypress. All of their coffins were made of the richly fragrant redwood – which meant this was a highly revered product. We also know in Turkestan, a very compact version of the Cypress was planted to adorn cemeteries. It has very close affiliation with death and significance with man and God.

BIBLICAL REFERENCES TO FIR (LUMBER)

2 Samuel 6:5
1 Kings 5:8
1 Kings 5:10
1 Kings 6:15
1 Kings 5:34
1 Kings 9:11
2 Chronicles 3:5
Song of Solomon 1:17

FIR (TREES)

2 Kings 6:5
2 Chronicles 2:8
Psalm 104:17
Isaiah 14:8
Isaiah 37:24
Isaiah 41:19
Isaiah 55:13
Isaiah 60:13
Ezekiel 27:5
Ezekiel 31:8
Hosea 14:8
Nahum 14:8
Zechariah 11:2

FIR'S HEALING PROPERTIES

Several varieties of Fir oil are commonly used in aromatherapy. *Abies alba*, or Silver Fir, is a species of Fir tree native to Europe.

Fir's viscous essential oil is extracted from the needles, twigs or cones by a process of steam distillation. Its familiar, fresh, balsamic fragrance is similar to Pine, a fellow member of the Pinaceae family. With a scent that is evocative of Christmas time, Fir blends well with floral and fruity oils – such as Lavender, Rosemary, Cedarwood, Pine, Lemon, and Marjoram. As a middle note, it brings a sweet, woody scent to an aromatherapy blend.

TRADITIONAL USES

In Europe, Fir oil is traditionally prized for its fragrance and medicinal qualities. It was traditionally used to treat respiratory problems and muscular aches. *Abies alba* has the accolade of being the first species to be used as a Christmas tree, before becoming replaced by other types that are cheaper to cultivate or have denser foliage.

The Fir tree is regularly mentioned in the Bible. Interestingly, some believe the 'gold' brought by the three wise men was actually Fir oil. The mixture of chemicals contained in Frankincense, Myrrh and Fir oil, is considered to be the perfect therapeutic blend. At the time, essential oils would have been the primary source of medicine, so their gift was most likely to have been for therapeutic purposes.

MEDICINAL USES

Fir essential oil is refreshing and uplifting, with the ability to ease muscular aches and pains. It is also used to treat respiratory conditions, such as coughs, colds, flu, tonsillitis, and sinusitis. As an antiseptic, it is ideal for treating wounds, cuts, and burns.

Fir oil can help to decrease levels of cortisol, the 'stress hormone', in the body. Excess cortisol can lead to premature aging, thyroid dysfunction, blood sugar imbalance, high blood pressure and decreased immunity, among other things. It has been proven that just inhaling Fir essential oil can lower cortisol levels by around 25%.

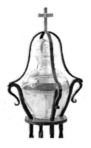

Frankincense

Along the southern tip of the Arabian Peninsula comes the most prized Frankincense in the entire world. Grown high up on the grid plateaus, Frankincense comes from a very low, twisted, bush-like tree that lacks a central trunk with it many prickly branches and pinnate leaves that extend every which way. Its sacred gum is obtained by slashing the roots and branches, making a deep incision and peeling back a narrow strip of its silvery bark, allowing the milky-white substance to ooze out. Once the air hits this substance, the sticky gum hardens into lumps. These lumps are either left on the tree for two weeks to dry or gathered and stored in mountain caves to dry for several months. Sap from the Frankincense plant is collected until the middle of September when rain showers end the harvest season.

Caravans of camels carried this precious and rare spice packed in sheep and goat skins in quantities of 20 to 40 pounds through the bleak Arabian Desert, west along the Red Sea coast – a trip that takes months. In the Red Sea regions, Frankincense is not only valued for its sweet odor when burnt but as a masticatory as blazing lumps of it are frequently used for illumination instead of oil lamps. Its fumes also serve as an excellent insecticide with its powerful bouquet, giving off no known toxicity.

Frankincense resins continue to be used for religious rites, medicines, and perfumes. When combined together with other spices such as Cinnamon or Cassia, they create a myriad of scents. Its fragrant smoke that burned in censors was offered to guests to make clothes, hair or beards smell pleasant. The sweet vapor dispelled the unwanted odors of unwashed bodies, as well as refuse in the streets. It also served as an insect repellent, warding off infestation from the many sacrifices and offerings. Today, Frankincense is collected for use in the home as incense, cosmetics and perfumes, refinishing varnish, and chewing gum.

In biblical times, Frankincense was used for religious ceremonies, and it was believed the prayers of the Cohanim (priests) for the people would ascend to heaven amidst the gentle wafts of incense. The Cohanim at the temple in Jerusalem burnt a kilogram of incense each day with their prayers. Exodus 30:34 records that

Frankincense was one of the elements used in the Holy Anointing Oil and was burnt with other substances during the meat offering as mentioned in Leviticus 6:15. In Leviticus 24:7 we read of how Frankincense was placed in purified form on the shewbread in the tabernacle. The giving of this incense to Yeshua at his birth has been interpreted as symbolizing his priestly office (Exodus 30:34; Leviticus 2:1, 15-16; Matthew 2:11). Historical documents reveal that the Queen of Sheba offered this prized aromatic gum to King Solomon. During Roman times, the Frankincense globules were worth their weight in gold.

Pure and holy sacred incense contains genuine Frankincense, which burns with ascending white smoke. Revelation 8:3-4 says that the original altar of incense continues to be used before the throne of God in Heaven.

Frankincense represents the godly prayers of his people rising to the throne (Exodus 30:1-9; Revelation 5:8). As ministers of the Lord, the priests burned incense before the ark in the Holy of Holies.

The Hebrew word *lebonah* means "incense," which is Frankincense. There are five other places in the Bible where *lebonah* was translated "incense" meaning "pure or white." This is because of the milk-colored drops of aromatic resin that flow from the slashed inner wood of the tree.

The *Boswellia olibanum* tree, which produces Frankincense, takes forty years to mature. In July 2006, the Tampa Tribune reported an over-harvesting of the trees and how the next generation isn't producing seedlings. The book of Revelation says that these oils will cease in the last days.

Pure Frankincense was also placed on the loaves of bread to symbolize the purity and fragrance of Christ, the true Bread of God (Leviticus 24:5-7, John 6:32-33, Exodus 30:34-36). A portion of this prescribed incense was not burned but merely placed before the ark in the Holy of Holies. God said that this is *where I shall meet with you; it shall be holy (the holiest) to you.* This represented the prayers in Heaven between Yeshua, God's Son, and the Heavenly Father.

In Numbers 16:46-50, it reads:

> *And Moses said unto Aaron, Take a censer, and put fire therein from off the altar, and put on incense, and go quickly unto the congregation, and make an atonement for them: for there is wrath gone out from the LORD; the plague is begun. And Aaron took as Moses commanded, and ran into the midst of the congregation; and, behold, the plague was begun among the people: and he put on incense, and made an atonement for the people. And he stood between the dead and the living, and the plague was stayed. Now they that died in the plague were fourteen thousand and seven hundred, beside them that died about the matter of Korah. And Aaron*

returned unto Moses unto the door of the
tabernacle of the congregation: and the
plague was stayed.

This incense used by Aaron in the book of Numbers stopped the plague from spreading. Believers can follow this example to protect themselves from the coming plagues in the last days.

Frankincense was not only used for incense but was offered as a gift. In Isaiah 60:3, Isaiah prophesied of the Magi's gifts: *And the Gentiles shall come to thy light, and kings to the brightness of thy rising.* And verse 6 continues, *The multitude of camels shall cover thee, the dromedaries of Midian and Ephah; all they from Sheba shall come: they shall bring gold and incense, and they shall shew forth the praises of the LORD.*

The Magi's arrival is seen in Matthew 2:11:

> *And when they were come into the house, they saw the young child with Mary, his mother, and fell down, and worshiped him: and when they had opened their treasures, they presented unto him gifts; gold, and Frankincense, and Myrrh.*

Mary and Joseph may have used the gifts to help protect Yeshua, keeping him strong and healthy.

A PURE CURE-ALL

The Egyptians considered Frankincense to be a universal cure-all, used for everything from gout to a broken head – in other words, from "head to toe."

In Northern Egypt, a sect of Jews called *Theraputei* continue to practice the healing arts by anointing the sick with oils and laying hands on them, as Yeshua did in his adult life.

BIBLICAL REFERENCES TO FRANKINCENSE

Exodus 30:34
Leviticus 2:1
Leviticus 2:15
Leviticus 2:16
Leviticus 5:11
Leviticus 6:15
Leviticus 24:7
Numbers 5:15
1 Chronicles 9:29
Nehemiah 13:5
Nehemiah 13:9
Song of Solomon 3:6
Song of Solomon 4:6
Song of Solomon 4:14
Isaiah 43:23
Isaiah 60:6
Isaiah 66:3
Jeremiah 6:20
Jeremiah 17:26

Jeremiah 41:5
Matthew 2:11
Revelation 18:13

FRANKINCENSE'S HEALING PROPERTIES

Used to treat every conceivable ill known to man, Frankincense resins and essential oil was valued more than gold during ancient times, and only those with great wealth and abundance possessed it. Researchers today have discovered that Frankincense essential oil contains sesquiterpenes, which help stimulate the limbic system of the brain (the center of emotions) as well as the hypothalamus, pineal and pituitary glands.

The hypothalamus, which is the master gland of the human body controlling the release of many hormones including thyroid and growth hormone, is now being researched in connection to how Frankincense effects it and its ability to improve the human growth hormone production as well as in the treatment of cancer.

Not only is Frankincense essential oil used for a variety of skin problems such as wrinkles, wounds, scars, dry skin, and relief for sore muscles, but there have also been some recent university studies showing the medicinal Frankincense essential oil benefits cancer as well as issues such as arthritis and anxiety.

Frankincense has been used in many cultures as incense because it was believed to produce a state of calmness. In 2008 scientists at Johns Hopkins University and the Hebrew University of Jerusalem found that there might actually be some truth to this, concluding that Frankincense does, in fact, relieve symptoms of depression and anxiety. The study, published in the May 20, 2008, issue of *FASEB Journal*, revealed that the positive effects were due to an element in Frankincense called incensole acetate. Gerald Weissman of the *FASEB Journal* remarked, "The discovery of how incensole acetate, purified from Frankincense, works on specific targets in the brain should also help us understand diseases of the nervous system."

This discovery of Frankincense as a natural remedy for anxiety and depression is very promising, but scientists are finding that it may have even more benefits than anyone realized. In 2006, the Virginia-Maryland College of Veterinary Medicine found that Frankincense helped reduce the size of skin cancer lesions on horses. John Roberts, director of the college's Center for Comparative Oncology, applied the Frankincense topically and found that the treatment eliminated small cancer cells and significantly reduced larger tumors. Roberts noted in his findings that this ancient medicine may have significant modern uses for chemotherapy of non-respectable malignancies.

Another study performed at the University of Oklahoma released data on the effects of Frankincense oil on bladder cancer cells. A study published in the journal *Complementary and Alternative Medicine* on March 18, 2009 revealed that Frankincense not only can differentiate between normal bladder cells and cancer cells but that it could also help inhibit cancer cell viability. The study stated Microarray and bioinformatics analysis proposed multiple pathways that can be activated by Frankincense oil to induce bladder cancer cell death.

The variability of the benefits of Frankincense oil is astounding. Not only is it being shown to have potential for reducing cancer cells, but another study shows that Frankincense extract from a particular variety of the Boswellia tree called *Serrata*, can relieve symptoms of osteoarthritis. Dr. Siba Raychaudhuri from the University of California Davis team noted that their team was concentrating on a particular ingredient in Frankincense called AKBA, which has been shown to have potent anti-inflammatory properties. The UC Davis team was testing this form of Frankincense because it has been proven to be highly effective without any of the adverse side effects other treatments possessed. Their research included a double-blind study with placebo controls and was performed on seventy patients. The team was hopeful after processing the results of their tests and commented that Frankincense was shown to have no major adverse effects in the osteoarthritis patients. It is safe for human consumption and even for long-term use.

TRADITIONAL USES

Frankincense is considered the Holy Anointing Oil of the Middle East and has been used in religious ceremonies for thousands of years. It has been used to treat every conceivable illness known to man, which caused it to be more valued more than gold in ancient times. Researchers today have discovered that Frankincense contains sesquiterpenes, which help to stimulate the limbic region of the brain, the hypothalamus, pineal, and pituitary glands. Frankincense is being used therapeutically in European hospitals and is being studied for its ability to improve the human growth hormone production.

Frankincense may help with allergies, asthma, depression, ulcers, snake and insect bites, bronchitis, cancer, respiratory infections, diphtheria, headaches, hemorrhaging, herpes, high blood pressure, inflammation, stress, tonsillitis, typhoid, and warts. Because it contains sesquiterpenes, it has the ability to go beyond the blood-brain barrier and helps to elevate the mind in overcoming stress and despair, as well as support the immunity system. It also increases the activity of leukocytes in defense of the body against infection.

MEDICINAL USES

Fumigation was one of the ways biblical people used essential oils – today, diffusers create the same effect.

Frankincense is safe to inhale, rub on the skin, and to take internally. It supports the immune system. The Arabs make teeth-whitening chewing gum from this resin. Frankincense heals cuts and wounds and also cures the common cold.

Today, Frankincense is used in many perfumes and colognes including the best-selling men's fragrance "Old Spice®" and Estee Lauder's "Youth Dew®."

Uses for this oil include asthma, headaches, hemorrhaging, high blood pressure, tonsillitis, warts, allergies, cancer, ulcers, bronchitis, and respiratory infections. Frankincense essential oil stimulates and elevates the mind. It overcomes stress and despair.

Frankincense is high in sesquiterpenes, enabling it to go beyond the blood-brain barrier. It increases the activity of leukocytes in defense of the body against infection. Frankincense also contains monoterpenes, which can reprogram cellular memory and promote permanent healing.

SPICE CHEST: DUTIES OF THE COHANIM

The Scriptures tell that the first healers and physicians of the Bible were the priests, who often anointed the sick and prayed for them. The role of the priesthood where they diagnosed, prescribed, and administered oils is described in Leviticus 13 and 14.

Their duties included: leading worship, receiving tithes, making sacrifices, and offering up prayers on behalf of the saints as spiritual counselors and hearers of confession. The Levites were to keep the fire burning day and night, taking care of the Temple of God. They mixed various oils for incense, healing, and anointing, and offered medical diagnosis and treatment. Their life was to exemplify righteousness.

The duties described for the priests in the book of Leviticus and in 1 Chronicles 9:26-30 actually describe the same responsibilities given to the Bride of Messiah, who is a priest as well.

1 Peter 2:9 says, *But ye are a chosen generation, a royal priesthood, an holy nation.* And Revelation 1:6 says, *And hath made us kings and priests unto God and his Father; to him be glory and dominion for ever and ever. Amen.*

As priests, followers of Yeshua must keep the fire in their hearts burning passionately for him and are instructed to pray for and anoint the sick, just as the Cohanim did.

The Bible says in 1 Corinthians 3:16, *Know ye not that ye are the temple of God, and that the Spirit of God dwelleth in you?* The body of a believer is the Temple of the Holy Spirit, and the believer is to keep his Temple – the body – attractive and in good repair. As a holy instrument, believers can anoint themselves to be sanctified vessels for God's use.

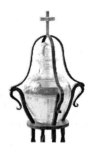

Galbanum

In Exodus 30:34-36 the instructions for the mixing of the holy incense are given:

> And the LORD said unto Moses, Take unto thee sweet spices, stacte, and Onycha, and Galbanum; these sweet spices with pure Frankincense: of each shall there be a like weight: and thou shalt make it a perfume, a confection after the art of the apothecary, tempered together, pure and holy: and thou shalt beat some of it very small, and put of it before the testimony in the tabernacle of the congregation, where I will meet with thee: it shall be unto you most holy.

The Old Testament Apocrypha dating back to 180 B.C. mentions the formula for holy incense in Sirach 24:15, 1,000 years after Moses.

Most of the spices and perfumes that made up the Temple incense were lovely and fragrant, but Galbanum had an earthier, parsley-like smell. The Jewish Talmud suggests that Galbanum – a less than wonderfully fragrant resin – was included in the holy incense because "every communal fast that does not include the sinners of Israel is not a fast."

The Hebrew word for Galbanum is *cheleb*, which means "the fat or the richest part." The Torah instructed the priest that when he offered up the goat as an offering made by fire for a sweet aroma, all the *cheleb* (the fat) belonged to the Lord and was forbidden for human consumption.

Believers are to be "lean" and to avoid fulfilling their lusts of worldly affections. The excess Yah gives a believer is to be offered back up to him to complete his mission and ministry on the earth, not for believers to be lazy and gluttonous with.

BIBLICAL REFERENCES TO GALBANUM

Exodus 30:34

GALBANUM'S HEALING PROPERTIES

Galbanum, which comes from the *Ferula galbaniflua* plant, has been used since ancient times by the Hebrew, Roman, and Greek cultures. It was used as incense, added to baths, applied topically as a skin balm, and worn as a perfume. Its fresh, earthy aroma helps to elevate the mind and spirit. Its chief chemical constituents are cadinene, cadinol, myrcene, and pinene.

Galbanum oil helps cure arthritis and rheumatism by improving blood circulation, due to its anti-arthritic and antirheumatic properties. It helps to heal old wounds like scars and helps to heal acne. It works well as a bug repellent due to the smell of the oil and repels parasites from humans and pets, like fleas, lice, and bedbugs.

TRADITIONAL USES

Galbanum was esteemed for its medicinal and spiritual properties as mentioned in Exodus 30:34. Egyptian papyri, as well as ancient Roman historians, record use of Galbanum for its antispasmodic, diuretic, and pain-relieving properties.

MEDICINAL USES

The essential oil of Galbanum is anti-infectious, anti-inflammatory, and analgesic. It supports the kidneys and a woman's menstrual cycle. It is also helpful for asthma, poor circulation, wounds, acne, bronchitis, cramps, indigestion, muscular aches and pains, nervous tension, scar tissue, and wrinkles. It may also help with abscesses, chronic coughs, cuts, inflammation, rheumatism, and stress.

Galbanum has been reported to bring harmony and balance, easing stress. It helps increase spiritual awareness and meditation.

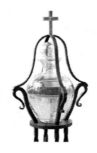

Garlic

Garlic only is only referenced once in Scripture, and yet, just its simplest mention brings a whole societal change into perspective. When the Israelites start to wane on their journey through the wilderness, they begin to crave meat. They cried, *We remember the fish we ate in Egypt at no cost--also the cucumbers, melons, leeks, onions and garlic.*

Allium sativum, the same garlic we know today, had been native to Asia and brought to Egypt by merchants. In her book *An Ancient Egyptian Herbal*, Lise Manniche describes how garlic has been found in Egyptian tombs and how Herodotus (484- 425 B.C.) proclaimed: "There is an inscription of Egyptian characters on the pyramid which records the quantities of radishes, onions and garlic consumed by the laborers who constructed it."

Interestingly, though, no such inscription has yet been found in a pyramid thus far! Since the Exodus is recorded to be some 480 years before the construction of the Temple of Solomon, which would place it around c. 1446 B.C., Herodotus speaks of a time almost a thousand years later.

Later, though, in 1922 when Carter opened the tomb of Tutankhamen, there were garlic cloves found on the floor. But, one has to ask, why were they there? So far no symbolic meaning has been attributed to garlic in the funeral process, so could it be that a workman dropped a little bit of his lunch?

In both ancient Egypt and ancient Greece, it became customary to feed laborers garlic, radishes, and shallots to build their stamina and strength. (Excavations show that the garlic may have been used as a very early performance enhancer at the first Olympic Games, too.) Roman soldiers took garlic into battle, but be very clear here: this was very much the food of the working class. The upper classes rejected it out of hand because of its fearful stench.

Here then, in Numbers 11:5, we see the very vivid image of the change of life these Israelites had endured. Toiling in the deserts of Egypt, life had been hard for Jewish slaves but to ensure the maximum productivity from the workforce, they had grazed on vegetables from the onion family. Now, here in the wilderness, that food source was gone. Life felt barren, different, and suddenly, not quite so appealing.

The Talmud, however, goes on to explain a little more about our understanding of the usage of garlic at that time. The Writings from the 2nd century details how people used garlic to get rid of infestations, be it insect or parasitic. It also explains how the bulb can be used to improve marital relations between a couple – in particular, one might presume this relates to fertility, but the meaning is not clear.

BIBLICAL REFERENCES TO GARLIC

Numbers 11:5

GARLIC'S HEALING PROPERTIES

Hippocrates, whom is considered the Father of Medicine, extols at length the virtues of using garlic during his practice. He described how it rid the body of parasites and insects as well as aided with digestion, in particular of fatty foods. He prescribed it for pulmonary and respiratory complaints, for abdominal growths, and, in particular, growths in the uterus. (One would suggest he means fibroids here.)

Fresh garlic (but not old or dried) has been found to be effective in the fight against E. coli.

Unlike most additions to the aromatic medicine chest, garlic really has no place in a body lotion or cream. Its pungent odor will always give it away. For this reason, only use the essential oil to combat very fierce attacks of fungal infections; its effects are swift, effective and offensive to the nostrils.

TRADITIONAL USES

In Ayurveda, garlic is considered to be a stimulant and thus an aphrodisiac. For this reason, ancient scriptures demand that it not be consumed by "monks, widows, adolescents or those who have taken vows." It is also used to treat bronchitis, dysentery, high blood pressure and tuberculosis in Asian countries.

Dioscorides, the physician to the Emperor Nero, was the first person to cite garlic as cleansing the blood. The idea still persists today and garlic is often used as a means to get rid of a cold or some types of stomach bugs.

In all ancient medicinal systems, there seems to be a common thread that it guards against evil, so we should also say "vampires" here!

MEDICINAL USES

Today garlic is a much-loved herbal medicine and addition to cuisine. It is thought that consumption of garlic can modestly reduce blood pressure and cholesterol. Garlic is also used to prevent some cancers and even to prevent atherosclerosis or congestion of the arteries.

Unlike most additions to the aromatic chest, though, garlic essential oil really is too potent to use aromatically. Its pungent odor will fill your house and last for weeks.

Emotionally, garlic is a warrior, but not a particularly nice one. It helps you to absorb your shadow side nature. This is particularly healing for people who are struggling to articulate hatred and rage effectively. This can be of specific use for people who are struggling to come to terms with the after effects of abuse.

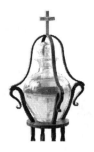

Henna

Henna, which comes from the *Lawsonia inermis*, is also known as Mehndi and referred to as "Camphire" (not to be confused with Camphor) in the Bible and comes from fragrant white flowers grown in clusters. Cyprinum is the name of the oil made from Henna flowers. It carries a delicate, sweet licorice note that creates a marvelous perfume with an orange tone. Henna Leaf Absolute is a very thick green paste described by some as a deep green herbaceous, tea-like bouquet. Henna Leaf Absolute is now mostly used for perfumes and biblical blends. It blends well with Neroli, Tonka Bean Absolute, Lavender, Blue Chamomile, Rose Absolute, Ylang Ylang and various spice oils.

In Israel, this treasured fragrance was used for skin aliments and to treat serious skin conditions such as leprosy and boils. In Egypt, it is rubbed over the body to keep cool. Henna played another important part of the Egyptian life as well. The scent of the Henna flower was thought to bring the dead back to life and was used on the skin to keep it soft and supple. In making a fashion statement, they used it to stain their nails red as well as other parts of the body. To not do so, one would be considered uncivilized and inferior.

In ancient times, a bride in the Middle East would apply this spice as a paste to her hands and feet the night before her wedding. This practice has begun to resurface as American brides decorate their body with temporary Henna art for their wedding. Today, Henna is commonly used for tattooing and is an important ingredient in Campho Phenique, an orangey red liquid used on minor cuts and scrapes.

Song of Solomon 1:13-14 says, *My beloved is to me a cluster of henna blooms.*

The Hebrew word for Henna (Camphire) is *kopher*, which means a ransom or price of life with its root word meaning "to forgive."

In the Middle East, a bride applies the spice of Henna as a paste to her hands and feet on the night before her wedding. This spice yields a red stain, which signifies the ransom of sinners through the shedding of Yeshua's blood on the tree.

In Isaiah 43:3 it says:

> *For I am the LORD thy God, the Holy One of Israel, thy Saviour: I gave Egypt for thy ransom, Ethiopia and Seba (Sheba) for thee. Since thou wast precious in my sight, thou hast been honourable, and I have loved thee: therefore will I give men for thee, and people for thy life.*

Think for a moment about what the hands and feet of our Lord did for us. His were stained with blood for the forgiveness of sins and as a ransom for his bride. For the believer, the hands signify work and the feet represent the way in which we walk. Our lives are to give forth the sweet fragrance of the Messiah's sacrifice on the tree as our ransom for sin.

1 Timothy 2:6 tells us: *Who gave himself a ransom for all, to be testified in due time.*

The way we walk and behave toward all men and our acts and deeds of charity emits a fragrance for the world to savor. In Ephesians 5:2-4 says:

> *And walk in love, as Christ also hath loved us, and hath given himself for us an offering and a sacrifice to God for a sweet smelling savour.*

The Scriptures go on to say what is a stench in the nostrils of Yahweh:

But fornication, and all uncleanness, or covetousness, let it not be once named among you, as becometh saints; neither filthiness, nor foolish talking, nor jesting, which are not convenient: but rather giving of thanks.

Through the triumph of the tree, Yeshua's resurrection gives us victory over the enemies of God (1 John 5:4, Hebrews 2:13). The bride price and ransom he paid was very costly and is represented by Henna, a most expensive spice.

In the Song of Solomon 4:12-14, the beloved responds to the Shulamite with these words:

A garden inclosed is my sister, my spouse; a spring shut up, a fountain sealed. Thy plants are an orchard pomegranates, with pleasant fruits; camphire, with Spikenard, Spikenard and saffron; calamus and Cinnamon, with all trees of Frankincense; Myrrh and Aloes, with all the chief spices.

Our garden is a private garden with walls, for him only. It is for his pleasure and his friends, the Heavenly Father, and the Ruach Ha Kodesh (Holy Spirit) to partake of our fruit, indicating the Messiah is being fruitful in our life. The Shulamite continues in Song of Solomon 4:16:

Awake, O north wind, and come, wind of the south; make my garden breathe out fragrance, let its spices be wafted abroad.

*May my beloved come into his garden and
eat its choice fruits!*

The Shulamite bride cries out to Yahweh to blow upon her garden. She feels confident he will be with her regardless of any situation she will face. Whether the circumstances are harsh (north wind) or pleasant (south wind), the bride's heart is to grow in maturity with her beloved, emitting a fragrance from her soul.

BIBLICAL REFERENCES TO HENNA (CAMPHIRE)

Song of Solomon 1:14
Song of Solomon 4:13

HENNA'S HEALING PROPERTIES

The word "Henna" is understood by many people around the world in many different ways. Most people associate Henna with dark-red/brown dye for hair and skin-tinting that is traditionally used in eastern cultures. The essential oil of Henna offers so much more.

TRADITIONAL USES

While Henna is commonly used as a dye for skin and hair, it is also used as an herbal treatment that has been widely accepted in the west, although it has been employed in eastern cultures for thousands of years, with its popularity beginning to spread. In Israel, this treasured fragrance was used for skin aliments and to treat serious skin conditions such as leprosy and boils. In Egypt, it is rubbed over the body to keep cool. Henna played another important part of the Egyptian life as well.

MEDICINAL USES

Henna essential oil is commonly used for its medicinal uses and contains a very high concentration of chemical components and nutrients. Some properties are antibacterial, antiviral, anti-inflammatory, hypotensive and many others. Many people think that the juice of the Henna plant is not very beneficial to health, but in fact, it can be directly applied to the skin for the relief of headaches.

It helps to bring down fevers according to Ayurvedic traditions. Although the antioxidant power of Henna has not been widely studied, the oil has been proven to be an astringent, which helps with anti-aging.

Henna oil has also been known to ease certain sleep disorders and promote better sleep.

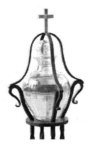

Hyssop

King David wrote in Psalm 51:7, *Purge me with Hyssop, and I shall be clean: wash me, and I shall be whiter than snow.*

David prayed this prayer after Nathan the prophet came and confronted him about his sin of going in to Bathsheba, committing adultery and murder in 2 Samuel 12:1-14.

As he began to meditate on the law, David felt great remorse and truly repented from his sin. His longing to restore his relationship with God reminded him of his understanding of the healing properties of Hyssop as a purifier and inspired him in his psalm of prayer to God.

The Hebrew word for "Hyssop" is *esob* and means "holy herb." Hyssop is considered to be spiritually purifying and serves as an aid in cleansing oneself from sin, immorality, evil thoughts, or bad habits.

The method of using of Hyssop oil (inhaled or applied to the body) to purge oneself from iniquity has scientific basis.

David Stewart, Ph.D., D.N.M. in his book *The Chemistry of Essential Oils Made Simple: God's love manifest in molecules,* he stated that Hyssop has constituents that can reprogram the DNA where sinful tendencies (negative emotions) are stored, thus releasing and cleansing the root cause of the action.

Another reason for the Jewish belief that Hyssop repels evil spirits is because of the passage in the book of Exodus, where Moses asked the elders of Israel to sacrifice a spotless lamb and to use a Hyssop branch to apply the blood of the lamb to the doorposts of their dwellings.

At the first Passover, the angel of death killed the firstborn son of every household except those whose doorway was marked with the lamb's blood using a Hyssop branch. Exodus 12:22 says,

> *And ye shall take a bunch of Hyssop, and dip it in the blood that is in the bason, and strike the lintel and the two side posts with the blood that is in the bason.*

Striking the doorposts would have released the scent of the Hyssop and the oil.

Yeshua, who died in his Bride's place, became the Passover Lamb. In John 19:29, it reads, *Now there was set a vessel full of vinegar: and they filled a spunge with vinegar, and put it upon Hyssop, and put it to his mouth.*

They dipped the sponge in sour wine or vinegar and extended it to his mouth on a branch of Hyssop because he is the door. This prophetic charade portrayed his blood as the only way of salvation and the Hyssop – symbolic of the Holy Spirit – as the one who purifies and sanctifies the believer.

BIBLICAL REFERENCES TO HYSSOP

Exodus 12:22
Leviticus 14:4
Leviticus 14:6
Leviticus 14:49
Leviticus 14:51
Leviticus 14:52
Numbers 19:6
Numbers 19:18
1 Kings 4:33
Psalm 51:7
John 19:29
Hebrews 9:19

HYSSOP'S HEALING PROPERTIES

The essential oil of Hyssop is extracted from the flowers and leaves of *Hyssopus officinalis*. Known in the ancient world as a holy herb for its purification abilities, this shrub grows mainly in the Mediterranean region.

TRADITIONAL USES

Hyssop is useful for easing fever, colds, and coughs as a decongestant. It helps reduce fat in tissue, raises low blood pressure, opens the respiratory system, and strengthens and tones the nervous system. Hyssop serves as a sedative and is good for quieting anxiety and clearing the mind.

MEDICINAL USES

For almost a millennium, Hyssop has been used medicinally for its antiseptic, disinfectant, and anti-infectious properties. It has also been beneficial for opening the respiratory system.

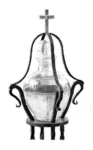

Juniper

The Juniper commonly found in the desert of Arabia rarely appears in the Bible. Scripture experts now agree the plant being referred to as Juniper was actually *retem* or the Spanish Broom, an enormous dense shrub with yellow flowers that grew very thickly in the water channels of the area.

The spiritual interpretations of the verses in which it appears, though, do in fact sit better with the old translations of the word. In some versions of 1 Kings 19:4, for example, the conifer has stood the test of time. 1 Kings 19:4 New American Standard Version calls it Juniper:

But he himself went a day's journey into the wilderness, and came and sat down under a juniper tree; and he requested for himself that he might die, and said, It is enough; now, O LORD, take my life, for I am not better than my fathers.

While the English Standard Version refers to it as the broom tree:

But he himself went a day's journey into the wilderness and came and sat down under a broom tree. And he asked that he might die, saying, It is enough; now, O LORD, take away my life, for I am no better than my fathers.

Somehow the imagery of the Juniper sits better.

In an ancient Apocryphal biblical text, a story relates how Mary and Joseph hid with the Christ Child under the branches of the Juniper to protect him from the onslaught of King Herod. If you have ever wondered how the infant escaped the genocide of the babies, it seems a Juniper tree may hold the key.

The verse cited above disclosed how the tree offered respite during Elijah's flight from Queen Jezebel and her hatred. The ancient Canaanites worshiped the Juniper as a symbol of their goddess Astarte. They believed it offered them fertility and protection.

The wood of Juniper, in itself, is not a very valuable commodity, except for the fact it burns incredibly hot. In Psalm 120:4, we read how the tribes sent scouts before the camels to find locations where the trees grew so that they could enjoy the best fires available to them. By night, the bush served as shelter from the wind and during the day served as shelter from the blazing sun. The Scriptures tell us in 1 Kings 19:4-5, that the prophet Elijah laid down and slept beneath this shrub on his journey from Beersheba.

In Job 30:4 it tells how when times were extremely hard the tree gave them food to eat.

Juniper berries are in fact cones, taking two years to mature on the branches. The Ebers Papyrus from 1500 B.C. revealed how ancient Egyptians used Juniper berries to dispel intestinal worms. If one considers how long sojourners roamed, perhaps eating undercooked or spoiled meat on days when food was lean, this could have been an extremely useful supplement.

Today, the berries are best connected with their flavoring of gin but are also used to improve the taste of many meats. They can be squeezed for their juices or used dried, much in the same way as peppercorns.

In his medieval herbals, Culpepper explains how the Juniper is known for its ability to contract the uterine muscles. Indeed, even today in some parts of Scotland, you might hear the catty remark that someone has given birth "over the savin," meaning they suspect the mother tried to induce a Juniper-fueled miscarriage.

During the Renaissance, Juniper was frequently used in art to represent chastity. For example, in Leonardo da Vinci's *Ginevra de' Benci*, not only was the subject named Juniper (*Ginevra* in Italian), but directly behind the portrait is a Juniper tree. The reverse of the portrait is decorated with a Juniper sprig encircled by a wreath of Laurel and palm that is memorialized by the phrase *Virtutem Forma Decorat* ("Beauty adorns Virtue").

Saint Juniper, "the Jester of the Lord," is sometimes called the saint of comedy. He was also known for his patience – it is said that St. Francis once described the perfect friar by citing "the patience of Brother Juniper, who attained the state of perfect patience because he kept the truth of his low estate constantly in mind, whose supreme desire was to follow Christ on the way of the cross." St. Frances held Juniper in such high regard he once said, "Would to God, my brothers, I had a whole forest of such Junipers."

BIBLICAL REFERENCES TO JUNIPER

1 Kings 10:4
1 Kings 19:5
Job 30:4
Psalm 120:4
Isaiah 41:19
Isaiah 60:13
Jeremiah 48:6

JUNIPER'S HEALING PROPERTIES

The refreshing scent of Juniper oil is said to have a cleansing effect on the mind and body. Its history dates back to the prehistoric times, with evidence of Juniper berries found at archeological sites in Switzerland.

There are several varieties of Juniper belonging to the Cupressaceae family. Originating in the southwestern USA, *Juniperus osteosperma* is commonly used in aromatherapy. The essential oil is extracted by steam distillation from the stems, leaves and flowers of the plant. As a top note, this oil has a clean, woody scent that is uplifting and revitalizing. It blends particularly well with Vetiver, Sandalwood, Cedarwood, Cypress, Pine, Fir and Lavender oils.

TRADITIONAL USES

In the Bible's Old Testament, a Juniper tree with an angelic presence sheltered the prophet Elijah from Queen Jezebel's pursuit. Similarly, a later apocryphal biblical account tells of how the infant Jesus and his parents were hidden from King Herod's soldiers by a Juniper during their flight into Egypt.

Since ancient times, Juniper has been used to treat urinary infections, headaches, respiratory problems, gout, and arthritis. It was also commonly used as a diuretic and aid for kidney and bladder problems.

The ancient Egyptians used Juniper to cure tapeworm, and since then it has been used to heal everything from tuberculosis to dysentery. As a purifier, Juniper was used in the ritual cleansing of temples. In the medieval era, families would hang bunches of Juniper over the doorframe to protect against witchcraft and evil spirits. In France, Juniper was often burned in hospitals to purify the air and boost immunity.

MEDICINAL USES

Juniper can be used to treat a range of respiratory conditions, including colds, coughs, flu, and infections. It has a refreshing aroma that can help to combat stress, depression, mental fatigue and anxiety. It is an excellent addition to skin care blends, particularly for dry, sensitive or aging skin. Juniper supports the urinary system, as well as boosting the circulation, digestive system and the elimination of toxins. Its analgesic properties can also help with rheumatic pain and cramps.

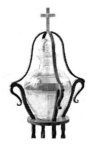

Marjoram

There is some debate as to whether Marjoram appears in the Bible or not. A quick glance would say no, but scholars now question the translation of the word we read as "Hyssop" (which, of course, is another of our beloved essential oils). It seems in some places a better translation is more likely to have been Marjoram.

Hyssop appears several times throughout the Bible. It is a plant held in high esteem and is cited as being present in some of the most important biblical events throughout history. When Moses regales the Ten Commandments to God's chosen people and also in his prescriptions to them about how to protect themselves at Passover, Hyssop is named as the herb in question. Most remarkably, too, in the New Testament, Hyssop is described in the story of the crucifixion, where a soldier gave Jesus a sponge and some Hyssop to drink. This image, though romantic and efficaciously sound (the high levels of ketones make spiritual transcendence far easier and would have been a superlative and compassionate choice to end suffering and help him to leave his mortal body behind), botanically, it seems unlikely that this could have been so.

Hyssop has a flexible and spiky stem, and it is very rare that a specimen would grow to the length required for such an action. In Palestine, it is unlikely, since Hyssop is not a native plant of this area, hailing from the East Mediterranean and Southern Asia, in particular.

So what was this Hyssop, which was deemed so treasured?

In Hebrews 9:19, we see a similar disconnection between the description of what the plant was used for and the anatomical nature of Hyssop. *For when every commandment of the law had been declared by Moses to all the people, he took the blood of calves and goats, with water and scarlet wool and Hyssop, and sprinkled both the book itself and all the people.*

But the leaves of the Hyssop plant do not lend themselves easily to sprinkling (its form is similar to a cross between Rosemary and Lavender), and so scholars proclaim that the Arabic term *zat'ar* refers instead to the family containing Marjoram or Thyme, and this is a more likely proposed translation.

In 1 Kings 32, we hear in praise of Solomon: *He could speak with authority about all kinds of plants, from the great cedar of Lebanon to the tiny Hyssop that grows from cracks in a wall. He could also speak about animals, birds, small creatures, and fish.* A wise and knowledgeable king would not make such a fundamental error in describing Hyssop as "springing from a wall" because it does not. This is not an apt description of Hyssop's growing habits at all, but it is a good description of a very specific type of Marjoram, *Origanum maru*, which particularly thrives growing on terraces and out of walls.

But Marjoram would not fit the translation of the plant from the crucifixion, and however as much as the idea that the herb used to ease Christ's pain was Hyssop, it seems likely that the correct attribution of the word would be *hussopo* (not Hyssop), which actually means "javelin" and thus a sponge of vinegar was given to the Lord on a javelin.

BIBLICAL REFERENCES TO MARJORAM

Exodus 12:22
Leviticus 14:4
Leviticus 14:6
Leviticus 4:9
Numbers 19:6
Numbers 19:18
1 Kings 4:33

Psalm 51:7
John 19:29
Hebrews 9:19

MARJORAM'S HEALING PROPERTIES

Marjoram is a nervine tonic and helps to balance the central nervous system (CNS), which makes it very useful if stress is a cause in triggering certain symptoms such as insomnia and migraines, for example. Its properties include being antispasmodic, nervine and carminative as well as being cephalic. Conditions such as stomach and leg cramps all benefit from its antispasmodic action.

It is a carminative plant and so balances and relaxes the digestive tract. Sufferers of diarrhea or constipation, as well as heartburn, indigestion, nausea or even belching, find relief from this plant. Marjoram is also very useful for bronchial asthma or coughs as it helps to relax these tissues, too. The essential oil is very gentle and is of particular help for children with coughs and runny noses; even when used in an evaporator or diffuser, its strength is enough to bring about a gentle sleep.

This same antispasmodic action makes Marjoram an excellent choice for muscle rubs. It's great for use on muscle pain and rheumatic aches, particularly because of its warming quality to circulation, or perhaps opt for it in rubs for athletic and sports preparations.

Interestingly, in studies into cultural differences in women's experiences of menopause, it has been identified that in some areas of rural Greece (as well as Mayan women) they suffer no symptoms at all. Could this be attributed to the Marjoram tea, which is their traditional remedy to aid the onset of menopausal symptoms? Certainly, the essential oil is beautifully used in abdominal massage oils when there is an absence or irregularity of menses. One has to wonder if this might also be thanks to the soothing CNS mechanism, too.

TRADITIONAL USES

Marjoram is a much under-used herb today, but historically it played a large part in Greek medicine. Traditionally the herb, known as "Joy of the Mountains," was associated with Aphrodite it was included in love potions and elixirs. Often, it would be used in wedding bouquets and bridal headdresses in Greece to sanctify wedded bliss.

In traditional medicine, there is a long-standing reputation that Marjoram growing in the garden would repel snakes. Even St. Basil mentions it in his Homily XI, *In Creation of Terrestrial Animals*, where he describes how animals understand the healing properties on a very innate level, thus: "You will also see the fox heal his wounds with droppings from the Pine tree; the tortoise, gorged with the flesh of the viper, finds in the virtue of Marjoram a specific against this venomous animal and the serpent heals sore eyes by eating Fennel."

MEDICINAL USES

The ancient Greek usage of Marjoram for wedded bliss exhibits a very different side of love from how we view it today, due to Marjoram's very specific anaphrodisiac property – that is, it curbs sexual desire. So here we see it used for platonic union of understanding and friendship. Today, this property is very useful for relationships enduring prolonged separations or to ease the emotional burden of a sexual veto for a while, perhaps post-natally, after trauma or because of sexual dysfunction.

It is a nervine tonic and also helps to balance the central nervous system (CNS), therefore, if stress is playing a part in triggering some symptom, then Marjoram is useful. Here we might think of insomnia and migraines, for example.

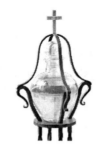

Mint

Mentha longifolia, commonly called horsemint, was native to Europe, Western Asia as far west as China and East to Nepal. In biblical times, it grew prolifically in Syria. It is suggested this was the Mint of biblical times and is a forefather of our own Peppermint.

Mint is mentioned in just one passage in the book of Matthew. The Pharisees are scolded by Jesus for religiously paying their tithes but not offering their inextinguishable love to God. The New American Standard Version in Matthew 23:23 says,

> *Woe to you, scribes and Pharisees, hypocrites! For you tithe Mint and Dill*

and Cumin, and have neglected the weightier provisions of the law: justice and mercy and faithfulness; but these are the things you should have done without neglecting the others.

Jesus' fury at the Pharisees lies in the fact they are so careful to pay their tithes to the temple with these herbs, but when it comes to offering something of real substance to God, such as their love, their commitment, and their trust, they are unable to take this step.

Tithes were commonplace to the Jews. There were tithes for everything. When you added them up, it would come to around 23% of a person's earnings. For a Pharisee, then, in Christ's opinion, this stopped short. Surely to be worthy of God's love, one must give everything he has, at least in his heart.

Any person who has a garden will know how prolifically Mint grows, too. It is a prolific plant, and while it had great significance to the Jews, it was by no means hard to come by.

One of the reasons it had originally been tithed to the temple was to help to cleanse it. Sprigs of Mint were strewn on the floor of the synagogue, releasing their vapors when a worshipper stepped on them. In a place where animals would be gathered to be slaughtered in sacrifice, this not only served as a balm on the fragrant air, but also releasing its precious molecules created a natural antiseptic.

The history of Mint's relationship with deities far predates the Bible. The ancient Assyrians burnt it on their altars to summon god in the fire, Nishku. Nishku was considered both heavenly as well as being terrestrial fire. He was seen as the intermediary between man and the gods since a burning sacrifice on the altar was believed to summon the gods. Burning Mint was their sweet request to speak with their deities.

The Egyptians and Greeks both flavored their foods and wines with the herbs. Mint was highly prized for its fresh aroma and sweet taste. For this reason, scholars speculate Mint was partaken with the bitter herbs of the Last Supper.

In the Middle Ages, people used powdered Mint leaves to brighten their teeth, and we see Mint cited in ancient Chinese medicals as early as the Tang Pen Tsao period c. A.D. 659.

It is believed the plant gained its name from the nymph Minta who appears in the myths of Persephone. The beautiful nymph captured the heart of Hades, who had abducted Persephone into the underworld. Jealous and incensed by this betrayal, Persephone turned the object of Hades' affections into a plant.

BIBLICAL REFERENCES TO MINT

Matthew 23:23
Luke 11:42

MINT'S HEALING PROPERTIES

Mentha Longifolia is a mint species of the Mentha genus, which is part of the Lamiaceae botanical family. It is sometimes referred to as Horsemint or Biblical Mint, on account of its references in the Bible. This species is native across Europe, Asia, and Africa, but extensively cultivated in the Holy Land region.

The essential oil is extracted from the aerial parts of the plant by steam distillation. As a top note, its aroma is fresh and minty, but milder than common Peppermint. Like other mint oils, it blends well with Eucalyptus, Lavender, Rosemary, Lemon, Basil and Benzoin.

TRADITIONAL USES

In the Bible, Mint was one of the herbs eaten with the Passover lamb. It was also tithed by Jewish leaders at the time, along with Rue and other herbs. Medicinally, *Mentha longifolia* has been used to treat respiratory ailments for hundreds of years. The leaves were infused to make a healing tea for coughs, colds, asthma, digestive problems, and headaches. Mint was also used to heal wounds and expel maggots. To disperse bees from beehives, Mint leaves were set alight to produce a pungent smoke.

MEDICINAL USES

Mint is predominantly used to treat problems of the digestive system, including cramps, gas, reflux, diarrhea, dyspepsia and flatulence. It soothes inflammatory skin conditions, such as eczema, as well as muscular aches and pains. Mint can be used to boost the circulation and help with respiratory problems, such as bronchitis. The cooling effect of Mint can also bring relief to headaches and fevers.

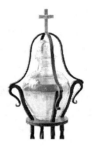

Mustard Seed

Brassica nigra has been cultivated across the Mediterranean and in Europe for thousands of years for its strong, tasty black seed.

The lowly Mustard seed plays an in important part in New Testament doctrine. It is mentioned in Matthew, Mark, and Luke as a favored simile in the parables told by Jesus about Faith and the Kingdom of God.

"As small as a mustard seed," was a common expression in the Jewish world, not least because of the vast proportions the plant could grow to. There are stories of men having been able to climb plants, which had grown to be trees with branches big enough to sit on. Other tales tell of soldiers passing under their boughs on horseback. These instances were, of course, rare, but it was common for a Mustard seed to grow to the size of a fruit tree. Certainly these trees had the capacity to rest birds in their branches.

Some Bible scholars suggest each of the stories mentioned in the Gospels may have referred to more than one specific instance of Christ's evangelism. Indeed, the passages are very similar. In Matthew 13:31 NASB, it reads,

> *In addition, he said onto them that another parable to them, saying, The kingdom of heaven is like a mustard seed, which a man took and sowed in his field.*

And in Matthew 17:20 NASB, it says,

> *And He said to them, Because of the littleness of your faith; for truly I say to you, if you have faith the size of a mustard seed, you will say to this mountain, Move from here to there, and it will move, and nothing will be impossible to you.*

In both Mark and Luke's Gospels, the Mustard seed is regarded as something that comes from man's heart (garden), such as an idea, ability or talent that if planted could easily yield significant benefits. In chapter 13 verse 19 it reads,

> *It is like a mustard seed, which a man took and threw into his own garden; and it grew and became a tree and the birds of the air nested in its branches.*

The results of exercising this talent are later revealed in Luke 17:6:

> *And the Lord said, If you had faith like a mustard seed, you would say to this mulberry tree, Be uprooted and be planted in the sea; and it would obey you.*

Understanding that the kingdom of God is not in a far-away place in the distance future, but is now and is within you, helps to grasp the verse in Mark 4:31 NASB:

> *And He said, How shall we picture the kingdom of God, or by what parable shall we present it? It is like a mustard seed, which, when sown upon the soil, though it is smaller than all the seeds that are upon the soil, yet when it is sown, it grows up and becomes larger than all the garden plants and forms large branches; so that the birds of the air can rest in its shade.*

At closer inspection, there is a yet another allegory at play when Christ refers to his tiny devout band of followers. How can such a marginal faction have power over the religions of the East? Their number might be few, but their faith is strong and resilient and has the power to change the world. The early-day church believers were that tiny but steadfast Mustard seed.

BIBLICAL REFERENCES TO MUSTARD SEED

Matthew 13:31
Matthew 17:20
Mark 4:31
Luke 13:19
Luke 17:6

MUSTARD SEED'S HEALING PROPERTIES

Although not commonly used in aromatherapy today, Mustard seed oil has a long history of traditional use across Asia. Unlike the fatty vegetable oil produced from Mustard seeds, the essential oil is highly toxic and should be used with caution.

Mustard seeds are ground and macerated in water, and then distilled to extract the pure essential oil. With a pungent, bitter scent, Mustard seed essential oil contains at least 92% allyl isothiocyanate. As well as Mustard, this chemical is also responsible for the distinctive taste of horseradish, radish and wasabi, which are fellow members of the Brassicaceae family. For aromatherapy purposes, Mustard seed oil does not blend particularly well with any other essential oil, due to its overpowering odor.

TRADITIONAL USES

In India, Mustard seed oil has been used as a traditional remedy for digestive problems for thousands of years and is still sometimes used today. Throughout history, Mustard seed oil has featured in eastern and western medicine.

In the Canonical gospels of the Bible, Jesus explained the concept of faith using the parable of the Mustard seed – which, despite being "smaller than all other seeds" eventually grows into a tree large enough for birds to nest in its branches.

The Mustard seed has symbolic significance to many of the world's major religions. It features in a famous Buddhist fable that teaches the reader not to wallow in grief, but to accept that death is an inevitable part of life. Jewish texts compare our universe to the size of a Mustard seed, to represent the insignificance of our world on Earth. The Quran frequently uses the Mustard seed to represent something minuscule in size, such as its explanation that "a deed even as small as a mustard seed one will duly be recompensed."

MEDICINAL USES

Mustard seed oil is warming and stimulating, which can help with digestive problems, muscular aches, and respiratory conditions. It is used to treat colds, chills, fevers, chilblains and all types of aches and pains. In the east, Mustard seed oil is also used to promote hair growth and inhibit fungal and bacterial infections.

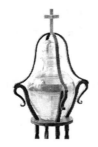

Myrrh

Commiphora myrrha, a shrub that produces Myrrh, can grow up to 30 feet in height. The trunk exudes a natural oleo resin that hardens into what is classified as reddish-brown tears. Native collectors make incisions into the trees in order to increase their yield. Myrrh has been used for centuries as an ingredient in incense, perfumes, and for embalming and fumigation in ancient Egypt.

Rich with symbolism, Myrrh is mentioned numerous times in the Bible. It is the first oil described in the Bible in Genesis 37:25, when Joseph's jealous brothers sold him into slavery to a caravan of Ishmaelites (incense traders) who were on their way to Egypt, carrying "balm and

Myrrh." Years later during the famine, Joseph's brothers came to Egypt to buy food, encountering Joseph as an Egyptian prince.

Interestingly, their father Jacob, (now called Israel) told his sons to take gifts for the prince. The Scripture says they brought Joseph balm and Myrrh (Genesis 43:11) – the same two oils that accompanied Joseph into slavery.

Not only is Myrrh the first oil mentioned in the Bible, it is the last one referred in Revelation 18:13:

And Cinnamon, and odours, and ointments ("Myrrh" in the Greek), *and Frankincense, and wine, and oil, and fine flour, and wheat, and beasts, and sheep, and horses, and chariots, and slaves, and souls of men.*

As the last oil mentioned in Revelation 18:13, it describes the destruction of Babylon when all of these fragrances and ointments will be no more.

The Greek word for Myrrh is *smurna*, which shares the same root name of the city and church mentioned in the book of Revelation. Smyrna was the second church of the seven churches of Asia John was instructed to write in Revelation 2:8-11. Interestingly, this church was distinguished as being persecuted and understood the bitterness of mistreatment for the sake of the Gospel.

Myrrh was one of the first gum resins/oils given as a gift to Yeshua as a young child by the Magi in Matthew 2:11. It was also the last oil offered to Yeshua at Golgotha when he was crucified. In Mark 15:23, it says, *And they gave him to drink wine mingled with Myrrh: but he received it not.*

SPICE CHEST: PREPARATION WITH MYRRH

In Esther 2:12, the Bible describes Esther's preparations for becoming queen which involved six months with the oil of Myrrh, a spice commonly used in preparing bodies for burial.

A similar custom is described in the Song of Solomon revealing another bridal tradition concerning the use of Myrrh. In the Song of Solomon 1:13, the bride responds to the king and says, *A bundle of Myrrh is my wellbeloved unto me; he shall lie all night betwixt my breasts.* This reflects a popular custom of laying a bundle of Myrrh on one's chest while sleeping as a beauty treatment in preparation for a wedding. Both of these examples from the Word teach believers that the first step to becoming the Bride of Messiah is to spiritually put the flesh to death.

Most believers know from experience the works of the flesh are the first issues God deals with when they come to know Yeshua as their Savior.

The Scriptures list these works in Galatians 5:19-21:

> *Now the works of the flesh are manifest, which are these;*

> *Adultery, fornication, uncleanness,*
> *lasciviousness, idolatry, witchcraft,*
> *hatred, variance, emulations, wrath,*
> *strife, seditions, heresies, envyings,*
> *murders, drunkenness, revellings,*
> *and such like: of which I tell you*
> *before, as I have also told you in time*
> *past, that they which do such things*
> *shall not inherit the kingdom of God.*

Esther didn't do it alone, as scripture shows. She had the king's eunuch Hegai to guide her in how to prepare. Believers also have a guide – the Holy Spirit – showing them all things in how to ready themselves for his return.

In the same way Esther prepared, the Spirit provides his betrothed ones with oil of Myrrh, which represents the fellowship of his sufferings, being conformed to his death. Philippians 3:10-11 reads,

> *That I may know him, and the*
> *power of his resurrection, and the*
> *fellowship of his sufferings, being*
> *made conformable unto his death; if*
> *by any means I might attain unto the*
> *resurrection of the dead.*

Because of what Yeshua did, the Lord's Bride can share in his victory over sin, the world, and the flesh. The Scriptures also tell us to rejoice in these trials. Colossians 1:24 says,

> Who now rejoice in my sufferings for you, and fill up that which is behind on the afflictions of Christ in my flesh for his body's sake, which is the church.

The Bible assures the believer that when the Messiah returns for his bride, we will actually smell his coming because his garments have been soaked in these fragrances in the midst of the throne room. Revelation 8:3-4 tells us that the original altar of incense continues to be used before the throne of God in Heaven. Psalm 45:8 describes Yeshua's garments: *All thy garments [smell] of Myrrh, and Aloes, [and] Cassia, out of the ivory palaces, whereby they have made thee glad.*

These spices are emitted in our lives when we clothe ourselves with righteous acts and deeds as the Bride of Christ and spend quality time with him. People will begin to recognize there is something different about you when you have been in his presence. Hebrews 1:8-9 affirms that this psalm refers to the marriage of Yeshua.

TEARS OF MYRRH

During the Messiah's final agonizing hours in the Garden of Gethsemane, the weight of the world's sins crushed the Savior like a wine press, causing him to sweat great tears of blood.

His bitter sufferings can be compared to Myrrh, a highly prized spice used in perfumes and incense, extracted by piercing the tree's heartwood and allowing the gum to trickle out and harden into bitter, aromatic red droplets called "tears." The Hebrew word for Myrrh (Strongs #4753) is *mowr*, which means "distilled" and comes from the root word *marar*, which means "bitterness."

After the Savior's crucifixion, his body was prepared with Myrrh. As a member of Yeshua's body, believers are to be made ready with the burial of their sins at the cross. They must die to the old life as death is the first step in preparation for those who will become the Bride of the Messiah.

Yeshua told his disciples in Matthew 16:24b-25, *If any man will come after me, let him deny himself, and take up his cross, and follow me. For whosoever will save his life shall lose it: and whosoever will lose his life for my sake shall find it.*

As joint heirs with the Messiah, his Bride is to share in his affliction according to 2 Corinthians 1:5, so that she can be triumphant through the bitterness of suffering. Believers are told to rejoice in this. Colossians 1:24 says, *Who now rejoice in my sufferings for you, and fill up that which is behind of the afflictions of Christ in my flesh for his body's sake.*

Myrrh is a fixing or servant oil which is used by apothecaries to enhance the fragrance of the other oils and make them last longer. Isn't that just like the Messiah? He is a servant and desires to lift up his Bride and enhance her with beautiful things.

BIBLICAL REFERENCES TO MYRRH

Genesis 37:25
Genesis 43:11
Exodus 30:23
Exodus 30:34
Esther 2:12
Psalm 45:8
Proverbs 7:17
Song of Solomon 1:13
Song of Solomon 3:6
Song of Solomon 4:6
Song of Solomon 4:14
Song of Solomon 5:1
Song of Solomon 5:5
Song of Solomon 5:13
Matthew 2:11
Mark 15:23
John 19:39

MYRRH'S HEALING PROPERTIES

Aromatherapists use Myrrh as an aid in meditation or before healing. Its actions are characterized as the following: antimicrobial, antifungal, astringent, healing, tonic, stimulant, carminative, stomachic, anticatarrhal, expectorant, diaphoretic, vulnerary, locally antiseptic, immune stimulant, bitter, circulatory stimulant, anti-inflammatory, and antispasmodic.

Its warm, balsamic odor with sweet and amber tones falls into the category as a base note. It is known as a fixing oil and servant oil, as it enhances the fragrance of other oils.

TRADITIONAL USES

Middle Eastern people have used Myrrh essential oil for skin conditions, such as cracked or chapped skin and wrinkles. Myrrh essential oil has commonly been used in oral hygiene products. In folk tradition, it was used for muscular pains and in rheumatic plasters.

Called *Mo Yao* in China, it has been used since at least 600 B.C. primarily as a wound herb and blood stimulant. Gerard said of Myrrh, "the marvelous effects that it worked in new and green wounds were here too long to set down…" Myrrh oil, distilled from the resin, has been used since ancient Greek times to heal wounds.

In biblical times, Myrrh was used on pregnant mothers for protection against infections and to elevate feelings of wellbeing. During labor, Myrrh was massaged on perineum to facilitate stretching. After childbirth, it was used to prevent abdominal stretch marks. It was customarily used on newborn umbilical cords to protect the naval from infection. Other uses in ancient times included: skin conditions, oral hygiene, embalming, and as an insect repellent. As a fixing oil, it enhanced the fragrance of other oils making their fragrance last longer.

MEDICINAL USES

Myrrh was known to act as a pain-reliever, which is why the Romans mixed it with the sour wine and offered it to Yeshua on the cross. Recent studies and medical research has discovered that Myrrh is anti-infectious, antiviral, antiparasitic, hormone-like, anti-inflammatory, and antihyperthyroid. It soothes skin conditions and supports the immune system.

Dr. Mohamed Rafi at Rutgers University discovered Myrrh to be anti-cancer and effective for prevention and treatment of breast and prostrate cancer, according to the *Journal of Natural Products*. Other uses include treating bronchitis, diarrhea, dysentery, hyperthyroidism, stretch marks and skin conditions, eczema, gingivitis, gum infections, asthma, athlete's foot, thrush and vaginal thrush, ulcers, and viral hepatitis. *Nature* magazine reported in an article entitled "Analgesic Effects of Myrrh" that Myrrh promotes a feeling of security. Many find just inhaling the fragrance lifts the spirit.

It contains sesquiterpenes, enabling it to go beyond the blood-brain barrier. It increases the activity of leukocytes in defense of the body against infection. Myrrh essential oil constituents have a direct effect on the hypothalamus, pituitary, and amygdale, the seat of our emotions.

It helps support the immune and endocrine system. Other uses include: Candida, coughs, digestion, fungal infection, hemorrhoids, mouth ulcers, ringworm, sore throats, skin conditions such as wounds, cracked skin and wrinkles.

SPICE CHEST: HOW ESSENTIAL OILS WORK

Using therapeutic grade essential oils on a daily basis can keep the body healthy, prevent disease, and even reverse damage.

Research has shown that the number one cause for depression is the loss of oxygen around the pineal and pituitary glands. They have also discovered that with careful application of essential oils to the soles of the feet, it enables the oil to reach every cell in the body within 20 minutes. This may be why people in biblical times lived so long.

Principal essential oils contain various constituents, including these three compounds: phenylpropanoids, sesquiterpenes, and monoterpenes. These three constituents are unique to essential oils and are produced naturally by the plant with the intelligence and capacity to do the following:

- **Phenylpropanoids** - cleanse the receptor sites
- **Sesquiterpenes** - erase the incorrect information in the DNA or cellular memory
- **Monoterpenes** - reprogram the cellular intelligence back to God's original plan with correct information

Sesquiterpenes carry oxygen to the brain and stimulate the pineal and pituitary glands. Three of the four oils in the world with the highest known concentration of sesquiterpenes are biblical oils: Cedarwood, Sandalwood, and Spikenard.

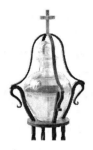

Myrtle

Myrtus communis, Myrtle essential oil, comes from a small tree grown now in France with many tough, slender boughs. It has a brownish-red bark with small pointed leaves. It produces flowers, which turn into black berries; both the flowers and leaves are very fragrant.

The Hebrew word *Hadassah*, Esther's Hebrew name, means "Myrtle." Because the Bible mentions this, she may have used Myrtle during her preparation for its therapeutic qualities of balancing the hormones. In Esther 2:7 it says:

> *And he brought up Hadassah, that is,*
> *Esther, his uncle's daughter: for she had*

neither father nor mother, and the maid was fair and beautiful; whom Mordecai, when her father and mother were dead, took for his own daughter.

Myrtle is also a treasured herb used in the celebration of the Feast of Tabernacles as seen in the Feast of Sukkot in Nehemiah 8:15 and Zechariah 14:16. Myrtle (Strongs #1918) is a picture of Elohim *echad*, as seen in Deuteronomy 6:4:

> *Hear, O Israel: The LORD our God is one LORD.*

Its leaves are in clusters of groups of threes, but all grow from the same point on the stem. The Hebrew word *echad* means "one comprised of more than one." The leaves of the Myrtle plant are a picture of the Father, Son, and Ruach HaKodesh – the Holy Spirit – as it says in Deuteronomy 6:4.

BIBLICAL REFERENCES TO MYRTLE

Nehemiah 8:15
Isaiah 41:19
Isaiah 55:13
Zechariah 1:8
Zechariah 1:10
Zechariah 1:11

MYRTLE'S HEALING PROPERTIES

The ancient Egyptians used Myrtle, a plant native to Africa, to remedy sore throats and coughs. As early as 1867, evidence shows that the essential oil was commonly being used by medical practitioners.

TRADITIONAL USES

Research on Myrtle has been done for normalizing hormonal imbalances of the thyroid and ovaries, as well as balancing the hypothyroid. It has also been researched for its soothing effects on the respiratory system.

MEDICINAL USES

Myrtle essential oil has common use as an astringent, antiseptic, vulnerary, bactericidal, expectorant and decongestant. Aromatherapy applications include usage to combat sore throats and coughs.

The therapeutic properties of Myrtle show that it is anti-infectious, a liver stimulant, eases prostate, is a decongestant, and a skin tonic. It is a light antispasmodic, hormone-like for the thyroid and ovary, and also serves as a tonic for the skin.

Myrtle has been used to help with asthma, sinus and respiratory infections, tuberculosis, hormone imbalances, and hypothyroidism.

Other uses include bronchitis, coughs, insomnia, respiratory tract ailments, and sinus infection. Myrtle has also been used for anger, asthma, cystitis, diarrhea, dysentery, dyspepsia, flatulence, hemorrhoids, infectious diseases, pulmonary disorders, skin conditions such as acne, blemishes, bruises, oily skin, psoriasis, and sinusitis. Its fragrance has been known to be elevating and euphoric. Myrtle is very helpful for clearing anger.

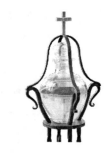

Pine

The Pine tree is mentioned many times throughout the Bible; however, there are so many references to Fir, Cypress, and Juniper, it could be that each tree is interchangeable. Particularly on Mount Lebanon, there are many differing species of Pine growing. Most notable of these is the largest, the *Sunobar kubar* found growing on Palestine's sandy plains. Its wood is widely used in construction to build beams and rafters of buildings.

In some ways tracing the history of the conifers through the Bible can be problematic as translation can be ambiguous. In Nehemiah 8:15, a tree of resinous nature is translated as Pine in the King James Version:

And that they should publish and proclaim
in all their cities, and in Jerusalem, saying,
Go forth unto the mount, and fetch
Olive branches, and pine branches, and
Myrtle branches, and palm branches, and
branches of thick trees, to make booths, as
it is written.

Compare this translation with the NIV verse of Nehemiah 8:15:

And that they should proclaim this word
and spread it throughout their towns and
in Jerusalem: Go out into the hill country
and bring back branches from Olive and
wild Olive trees, and from Myrtles, palms
and shade trees, to make booths--as it is
written.

We see this trend repeatedly with Pine, creating a source of great debate. Some suppose the Hebrew word *ets shemen* might be better interpreted as elm, others say oak, or holm, or ilex. Its best literal translation is "Fat wood tree," which, of course, could just as likely pertain to Olive's heavy oil content, but most scholars agree Pine is correct.

The main part of the argument for the references pertaining to Pine is how plentifully two species, in particular, flourish in Palestine and Lebanon. These are *Pinus pinea*, the Stone pine, and *Pinus halepensis*, the Alleppo pine. High up in the mountains overlooking the sea, their heady scent penetrates the heated air. Two more references show just how very revered the Pine was. Isaiah 41:19 states,

> I will put Cedar, Acacia, Myrtle, and oil trees in the wilderness. I will set Fir trees, Pine, and box trees together in the desert.

And, in Isaiah 44 verse 14 it says,

> When he heweth him down cedars, he taketh also a holm-oak and a terebinth he chooseth for himself among the trees of the forest: he planteth a pine, and the rain maketh it grow.

WAS NOAH'S ARK MADE OF PINE?

In Genesis, we read how God told Noah to build an ark (an enormous box-shaped vessel) of "gopher wood." God said: *Make thee an ark of gopher wood* (6:14). This is the only place this strange wood is mentioned. Cypress wood may have been the wood used.

However, in a 16th century Geneva, gopher wood was nominated as being Pine trees. Worried about this strange translation once the King James Version was printed, Pine had been returned to Gopher, with no translation risked.

The 1978 the New International Version ventured a little more courageously and asserted Gopher was, in fact, Cypress. The Jewish Encyclopedia states identification of gopher with Cypress is "arbitrary and unsatisfactory" and continues that this classification "rests on the mere assumption that the roots of these two words are akin. According to P. de Lagarde, gofer has been shortened from *gofrit*, which originally meant Pine, from old Bactrian *vohukereti*, and then later also Sulphur. This is attributed to the similarity in appearance sulfur bears to pine-resin."

SO WHY WAS PINE SO LOVED?

A far older translation of the verse throws beautiful, dappled sunlight on our quest to understand this tree.

The commentary by Metzudat David ("The Bulwark of David") gives us: "There is the man who will take Cypress or oak because these trees are more beautiful and because they are not as strong as cedar he reinforces them with nails of the forest trees. He planted a Pine. That is to say, there is one who will bother even more and from the start plants a Pine that is good for the job and waits until it grows and will be worthy of a statue and rain and will grow. As if saying that it is the intention of the planter to make a statue out of it…"

THE BEAUTIFUL PINE TREE

Pine is one of the strongest, fastest-growing wood sources, but clearly someone who was determined to make something wondrous must invest in their quest. It is known throughout the world for its ability to grow tall and very straight. Today, more than half the world's construction is built using Pine. These properties would have held the same value thousands of years ago.

Pinus hapiensis in particular can easily grow to 8 feet and if trees are given enough space to grow will reach far higher than that. The internal structure of the wood is laced with hundreds and hundreds of oil ducts, secreting resins. This means the wood is extremely volatile but is also very flammable. On the ancient sacred altars, priests would have strict codes about which woods to use and when. Their most favored were Pine, Fig, and Walnut because they burned so ferociously, sending clear messages of their intentions to God.

The leaves or needles of the Pine are extremely hardy. Growing in pairs around the branch, they can last for many years provided they have enough light. When they do fall, they create a majestic weed-oppressing carpet right over the ground.

SPICE CHEST: ANCIENT EGYPT'S KYPHI

Several ancient Egyptian Papyri mention Pine and Pine nuts (different tree) in their recipes for the ritual incense Kyphi. Initially, Kyphi (or you might also see it written as Kamet) was to clean and perfume the priests' temples before ceremonies. Later, the religious connotations changed and the Egyptians began to believe the smoke from the incense carried the prayers of the priests to the gods.

The first time we see it mentioned with religious attachment is in the Papyrus Ebers, dating back to the rule of Ramses VI in the 20th dynasty. It details a donation made by Ramses III of ingredients to makes kyphi for the temple at Edfu. Six ingredients were mentioned: Mastic, Pine resin (or wood), Camel grass, Mint, Sweet Flag and Cinnamon. Sadly the method of preparation or recipe did not survive for us to know, but it is suspected these might have been mixed with wine and honey, which would have to come from a different, more central source.

Edfu was built in the Ptolemeic dynasty in the 1st century B.C. where inscriptions remain on the walls detailing how other blends were created. The Mastic, Pine resin, Sweet Flag, Aspalathos, Camel grass, Mint, and Cinnamon are ground together in a mortar. Any liquid residue was then discarded. Cypress, Juniper berries, Pine kernels and a so-far unidentified plant material called Peker were then also ground and combined with the Mastic mixture. This powder combination was then moistened with a little wine and left to steep overnight. Raisins were then steeped in wine and combined with the mixture. For another five days, the mixture was left to steep so the properties and scents could marry and meld.

This delicious mixture was boiled and reduced by one fifth. Honey and Frankincense were combined and boiled together and also reduced by a fifth. Finally, the two mixtures were combined. Ground sticky Myrrh was then added to make the final mixture and form them into small pellets for burning.

The pinecone is an evolutionary precursor to a flower, hiding seeds between the segments of the cone. They are perfectly aligned with the series of the fibbonacci sequence and so have become part of history's sacred geometry and directly aligned to the pineal gland (*pineal* taking its name from the word pinecone). In the modern-day church, the cone has become the sacred symbol for illumination.

The pineal is considered to be the seat of enlightenment, the third eye, perhaps the seat of the soul. In Genesis 32:30-31 we see Jacob wrestling with God, and he sees him with his pineal. The literal biblical translation of the word "Peniel" means "Face of God."

And Jacob called the name of the place Peniel: For I have seen God face to face, and my life is preserved. And as he passed over Peniel the sun rose upon him.

We can trace the reverence of the pinecone back as far as the ancient Egyptians. Many artworks found in the tombs of ancient Egypt show the dead person entering the afterlife with a pinecone on their head. Interestingly, in his book *The Golden Bough*, James Frazer suggests there are depictions of Osiris, god of the dead and ruler of the underworld, being placed in the coffin carved out of a tree that looks like a Pine.

The staff of Osiris dating back to 1244 B.C. depicts two serpents spiraling around the staff to a pinecone. Nowadays it is suggested this portrays kundalini working its way through the chakras to the crown. This symbolism spans ancient Assyrian, Aztec, Hindu and Greek art.

The pinecone often depicts enlightenment and often it is paired with the serpent. It is interesting to see the two sides of fertility joined together, the serpent and her meaning of continual renewal alongside the pinecone. Many have suggested that in fact, then, the cone may have been the original translation of Eve's temptation, rather than an apple.

Followers of the ancient Greek god Dionysius carried with them wands topped with the cone, and similar symbolism is also found in druidic lore. Closer to our time, the cone resonates across the Catholic Church. The Vatican holds the cone in the highest of all esteems. The Pope himself carries a pinecone-topped staff. Consider, too, the Vatican's flag of the Holy See – not only does it contain the pinecone, but even the name Holy See seems to chime of the pineal. Outside of the Vatican in the Courtyard of the Pinecone, La Pigna holds precedence. The beautiful fountain which once oversaw Rome now greets visitors to the church's most Holy City.

SYMBOLISM OF PINE

The symbolism of this tree is diverse. It pertains to creativity, life, longevity, and immortality. In modern symbolism, the Pine tree is the symbol of festivity found on many Christmas cards, it but reaches back further through time, and it is well represented as the symbol of fertility. In the Bible, there are many allusions to the pinecone and it is synonymous with spirituality and communications with God.

BIBLICAL REFERENCES TO PINE

Nehemiah 8:15
Isaiah 41:19
Isaiah 60:13

PINE'S HEALING PROPERTIES

Out of over 175 varieties of Pine, *Pinus sylvestris* is considered to be therapeutically one of the safest to use in aromatherapy. Commonly known as Scotch Pine, the *Pinus sylvestris* accounts for around one-third of all Christmas trees.

Belonging to the Pinaceae family, this species is native to Europe and Asia. Its essential oil is extracted by dry distillation of the pine needles. The oil is usually clear or pale in color, with a fresh, woody balsamic scent that blends well with Cedarwood, Rosemary, Tea Tree, Lavender, Juniper, Eucalyptus, Lemon, and others.

TRADITIONAL USES

Pine has been in use since ancient times. The Egyptians used it in cookery while the Romans and Greeks used it therapeutically to treat muscular problems and respiratory conditions. In fact, Hippocrates – the founder of Western medicine – researched Pine as a remedy for muscular aches and pains. Since then, it has also been used to treat wounds, nervous exhaustion, and poor circulation. Native Americans would sleep on mattresses stuffed with Pine to deter lice and fleas. In Sweden, Pine needle tea is a traditional health drink, which is packed with vitamins and believed to fortify the system.

The Pine tree played a symbolic role in ancient pagan religions and was considered sacred in ancient Rome and Greece. Pine also had a strong Christian association and is mentioned several times in the Bible. It is no coincidence that the Pine tree came to be associated with Christmas time. This evergreen tree is thought to symbolize eternal life and God's everlasting love for humankind. Pine trees were plentiful on the Mount of Lebanon, and many believed they represent peace, joy or fertility.

MEDICINAL USES

Pine has similar therapeutic properties to Eucalyptus and is a popular oil to use in inhalations for all types of respiratory conditions. It has a strengthening effect on the body and can ease muscular stiffness, aches, and pains. Pine boosts the circulation and can help with disorders of the nervous system, such as neuralgia and fatigue. It can also help to treat urinary infections and skin problems, including cuts, sores, and lice.

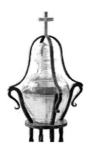

Olive Oil

Olive oil is an oil obtained from the Olive (*Olea europaea*; family Oleaceae), a traditional tree crop of the Mediterranean Basin. It is commonly used in cooking, cosmetics, pharmaceuticals, and soaps and as a fuel for traditional oil lamps. Olive oil is used throughout the world, but especially in Mediterranean countries.

The first recorded oil extraction is mentioned in the Hebrew Bible, which took place during the Exodus from Egypt, during the 13th century B.C. During this time, the oil was derived through hand-squeezing the berries and stored in special containers under guard of the priests. A commercial mill for non-sacramental use of oil was in use in the Tribal Confederation and later in 1000 B.C., the Fertile Crescent, and the areas consisting of present-day Palestine, Lebanon, and Israel. Over 100 Olive presses have been found in Tel Miqne (Ekron), where the biblical Philistines also produced oil. These presses are estimated to have had output of between 1,000 and 3,000 tons of Olive oil per season.

Dynastic Egyptians before 2000 B.C. imported Olive oil from Crete, Syria and Canaan, as oil was an important item of commerce and wealth. Remains of Olive oil have been found in jugs over 4,000 years old in tombs on the island of Naxos in the Aegean Sea. Sinuhe, the Egyptian exile who lived in northern Canaan about 1960 B.C., wrote of abundant Olive trees.

Olive oil is used as a carrier (vegetable) oil and the Bible clearly states that the only grade of Olive oil suitable for holy anointing purposes is the "first oil." The Bible discusses this in Leviticus 24:2:

> *Command the children of Israel that they bring unto thee pure oil Olive beaten for the light, to cause the lamps to burn continually.*

Today, the first oil is called "virgin oil." Virgin Olive oil has a wonderful fragrance and flavor and is not pressed from the fruit, but drained from the crushed fruit.

The "first oil" or virgin oil serves as a spiritual picture of the Bride of Messiah. She is the first to come out of Babylon on her own and is drawn by the Holy Spirit or

Ruach. The Bride has a fragrance the world recognizes as different.

The second oil, or "pressed oil," is inferior as its fruit is crushed, stamped, and squeezed to get every last drop of oil. This oil was not acceptable as an offering to the Temple, as it has no flavor or fragrance.

Believers who are sluggish and foolish have to be beaten and endure fiery trials like the "second oil" to come out of the world. The choice, of course, still remains theirs. Will a believer be a fragrant offering to him or be hard-pressed and remain tasteless to the world? 2 Corinthians 2:14-15 says,

> *Now thanks be unto God, which always causeth us to triumph in Christ, and maketh manifest the savour of his knowledge by us in every place. For we are unto God a sweet savour of Christ.*

BIBLICAL REFERENCES TO OLIVE OIL

Genesis 8:11
Exodus 27:20
Exodus 30:24
Leviticus 24:12
Deuteronomy 6:11
Deuteronomy 8:8
Deuteronomy 24:20
Deuteronomy 28:40
Judges 9:8

Judges 9:9
1 Kings 6:23
1 Kings 6:31
1 Kings 6:32
1 Kings 6:33
2 Kings 18:32
1 Chronicles 27:28
Nehemiah 8:15
Job 15:33
Psalm 52:8
Psalm 128:3
Isaiah 17:6
Isaiah 24:13
Jeremiah 11:16
Hosea 14:6
Amos 4:9
Habakkuk 2:19
Zechariah 4:3
Zechariah 4:11
Zechariah 4:12
Romans 11:17
Romans 11:24
James 3:12
Revelation 11:4

OLIVE(S)

Judges 15:5
Micah 6:15
Zechariah 14:4
Matthew 21:1

Matthew 24:3
Matthew 26:30
Mark 11:1
Mark 13:3
Mark 14:26
Luke 19:29
Luke 19:37
Luke 21:37
Luke 22:39
John 8:1

SPICE CHEST: WHAT IS A CARRIER OIL?

Carrier oils come from nuts, seeds or kernels that contain essential fatty acids, fat-soluble vitamins, minerals and other crucial nutrients. You will find a variety of carrier oils including Olive oil, Almond oil, and Pomegranate oil, each possessing different therapeutic properties. Distinct from essential oils, carrier oils do not contain aromatic scents (or only a very faint scent) and evaporate due to their large molecular structure. For this reason, most consider carrier oils are added as a vehicle for applying essential oils to the skin and do offer their own healing properties which essential oils do not possess.

OLIVE OIL'S HEALING PROPERTIES

Virgin Olive oil is an extremely versatile oil. It is a favorite on both dry and irritated skin with a light to medium green color and a rather heavy texture. It is very soothing and carries disinfecting and healing properties. Olive oil is quite legendary since it has been used over the centuries for multiple purposes, but due to its overpowering scent, this oil does not work well for massages. However, it is beneficial in some lotions for burns or scars. Olive is very beneficial for dry, damaged or split hair and is soothing to inflamed skin such as eczema. It has been proven to be very beneficial for rheumatic conditions and protects the body against harmful free-radical cell damage.

The "virgin" indicates it comes from the first pressing of the fruit. The "extra" means it comes from a single source.

TRADITIONAL USES

Historically, Olive oil has been the base for anointing oils. Olive oil is commonly used in body lotions, soaps and hair products. Olive oil has been used for stomach disorders, stimulates bile production, promotes pancreatic secretions and may even protect against stomach ulcers. Olive carrier oil can be used for many manufacturing applications though it may not be a preferred choice in any particular category.

MEDICINAL USES

Olive oil as a carrier has an appealing odor but can influence the smell of an essential oil blend. It will absorb into the skin although it can leave a slightly oily feel on the skin. It is considered non-toxic and non-irritant and can be used by anyone.

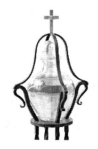

Onycha

Onycha comes from the Balsam or Benzoin Tree of the Far East. However, rabbis debate whether Onycha is a resin from a tree. Some believe it is an aromatic from a mussel or shell because of its Hebraic root. Others, such as Rabbi Gamaliel (whom the Apostle Paul studied under), believe it is actually a part of the balsam species.

The Hebrew word "Onycha" is *shecheleth*, which means "part of the holy incense, sweet kind of gum, and shines as the nail." Because of this definition, some believe Onycha comes from the same mussel that provides the purplish-blue color used to dye tzitzits or fringes on the prayer shawl.

As seen in Exodus 30:34, Onycha is used in the Holy Anointing Oil. It is also mentioned in the Talmud and the Old Testament Apocrypha.

According to Strong's Concordance, it is from the same root word as *shachal*, meaning "to roar; a lion from its characteristic roar." This describes Yeshua, the Lion of the tribe of Judah! The Lord has been given all authority in Heaven and Earth as the Lion of Judah (Matthew 28:18 and Revelation 5:5).

Mystery and debate surrounds what is known as Onycha. Some believe it to be of plant origin while others believe it to be from the finger-like operculum or the closing flap of certain snails. Rashi, a great Jewish scholar, believed Onycha to be a kind of root that grew from the ground. Some suggest it is extracted from *Styrax benzoin*, a type of resin used in the Tabernacle for incense in ancient biblical times.

The Encyclopedia of Bible Plants (F. Nigel Hepper, 1992) agrees that Onycha is more likely to be a plant resin. Rabbi Gamaliel believed it to be part of the plant species and said, "The balm of Onycha required for the incense exudes from the balsam trees." The Jewish Talmud, in which the Hebrew is of a later date than the scriptures, refers to the substance as *tsiporen*, which means "fingernail" and seems to be related to *sh'chalim*, meaning cress, a type of plant.

The Hebrew word for Onycha is *shecheleth* and refers to a resin with a nail-like shine, claw or hoof. For this reason, others believe it is an aromatic from the operculum of a shellfish, for example, the claw or nail of the strombus or wing-shell, a univalve common in the Red Sea (the same mussel from which the blue dye for the tzitzits (fringes) was obtained). The Greek word from the Septuagint 'onyx' also adds confusion. Onyx is an agate with a fingernail-like opacity that has for some reason been associated with a claw-shaped shellfish.

Tzori alludes to the Torah that it is a balm that brings healing to the entire body. Onycha was valued anciently for its ability to speed healing of wounds and to help prevent infection. The fragrance of Onycha is a reminder to Satan that he is a defeated foe and believers share in the Lord's authority "to tread on...all the power of the enemy" in his name (Luke 10:19).

BIBLICAL REFERENCES TO ONYCHA

Exodus 30:34

ONYCHA'S HEALING PROPERTIES

Onycha, a plant derivative, is highly aromatic and is credited as having great medicinal properties. It seems to be the most likely ingredient for the holy incense when considering the healing effect prayer has. Onycha is a very thick and heavy oil, which makes it impossible to pour.

Its scent will seem familiar to some because it contains vanillin aldehyde, which gives it a vanilla scent.

TRADITIONAL USES

Onycha was used for thousands of years for respiratory conditions. Onycha is valued for its ability to speed the healing of wounds and prevent infection with its antiseptic properties. Onycha is known by other names including "Friar's Balm," "Benzoin," and "Java Frankincense."

MEDICINAL USES

Healing properties of Onycha include anti-inflammatory, antioxidant, antiseptic and sedative. It combats arthritis, gout, asthma, bronchitis, and skin conditions. Other uses include arthritis, astringent, bleeding (slow or stop), chills, poor circulation, colic, cuts, deodorant, diuretic, expectorant, flu, flatulence, laryngitis, mucus, nervous tension, rheumatism, skin conditions such as chapped or inflamed skin, stomach, stress, urinary tract infection, and wounds. It's good for colds, coughs, and sore throats.

SPICE CHEST: ANOINTING THAT BREAKS THE YOKE

Psalm 133:2 describes the anointing of Aaron as: *precious ointment upon the head, that ran down upon the beard, even Aaron's beard: that went down to the skirts of his garments.* The words "precious" and "ointment" indicate that this was not just Olive oil but pure oils such as were used in the Holy Anointing Oil.

The Hebrew word for "anoint" is *masach*, which means "to smear, spread, or massage," and in some cases it means "to pour oil over the head or body." It shares the same root term as "Messiah," *mashiyach*, meaning "anointed one." In the New Testament, the Greek word *kristos* or "Christ" means "anointed one" and is used 361 times.

Other words and phrases used in the Scriptures such as anointing oil, ointment, spices, incense, perfumes, odors or sweet savors, aromas, and fragrances, all imply essential oils.

A unique act of anointing is found in ancient Chinese medicine – for thousands of years they have placed oil on the inside of the ear, and this place was called the *sheman* point. Yahweh instructed anointing this point of the right ear in Leviticus 14:17:

*And the rest of the oil that is in his
hand shall the priest put upon the tip
of the right ear of him that is to be
cleansed, and upon the thumb of his
right hand, and upon the great toe of
his right foot, upon the blood of the
trespass offering.*

This practice was used in a cleansing ceremony for leprosy to cleanse the leper and his house, and in another ceremony to release emotional patterns of guilt. Both of these rituals involved Cedarwood, Hyssop, and a "log of oil" (10 fluid ounces), which would have been beaten Olive oil containing aromatics. Modern research has found that this portion of the ear is where one releases and resolves issues of guilt regarding their parents.

The sacred act of anointing is mentioned 156 times in the Bible. The Hebrew word for "anointing" is *shemen*, which means "fat oil, fatness, or Olive oil." In Isaiah 10:27, it says,

*And it shall come to pass in that day,
that his burden shall be taken away
from off thy shoulder, and his yoke
from off they neck, and the yoke shall
be destroyed because of the anointing.*

It is the **oil** that breaks the yoke, not simply the act of anointing.

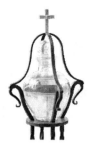

Pomegranate

Highly esteemed by Israelites, the Pomegranate was believed to be the original "forbidden fruit" in the Garden of Eden. It was also one of the seven species brought back by the spies to show how fertile the Promised Land was. Carved figures of the Pomegranate were principal ornaments adorning stately columns and pillars in Solomon's temple as well as worn on the High Priests' garments symbolizing life.

The Hebrew word for "Pomegranate" is *ramam or rimmon*, which means "to rise up" or "to be mounted up."

In Song of Solomon 4:3, Solomon describes his bride's *temples are like a piece of a pomegranate within thy locks.*

Solomon uses the Pomegranate theme for her temples to show fertility of the mind, where good seed is planted, and a harvest is sure. Her thoughts are on what is pure, lovely, and of good report. She is the true bride, with the mental state that matches the King's. Here the Holy Spirit finds a welcome depository for "things that are to come."

Here the words of Yeshua are quickly brought to mind. She has the mind of Christ.

The Pomegranate fruit, in relation to our temples, signifies that it is now the "fruit of the Spirit" that controls our lives (mounts or raises us up or above) rather than the lust of the flesh. The phrase "within thy locks" shows that she bears spiritual fruit that is veiled and hidden from the world for only the Lord to behold.

Some interpreters believe the reference to Pomegranates is a symbol of fertility. On a holy theme, greater significance might point to the use of the Pomegranate as it relates to the skirt of the high priest. At the bottom of the high priest's robe were Pomegranates interspersed with bells. With every step, the ringing of bells with the symbol for "fertility of life" bore witness to sight and sound to declare life. Life and abundance characterizes the Savior's bride.

The Pomegranate is native in regions ranging from Iran through the Himalayas in northern India. It was cultivated and naturalized over the Mediterranean region since ancient times. The Pomegranate plant is a neat, rounded shrub or small tree that can typically grow to 12 to 16 feet in height. Dwarf varieties are also known. It is usually deciduous, but in certain areas, the leaves will persist on the tree. The trunk is covered by a red-brown bark, which later becomes grey. The branches are stiff, angular and often spiny.

The Pomegranate's most famous and important appearance in the Bible is in Exodus. The Lord commanded Moses to make the roses of the Ephod and embroider them with many colored Pomegranates. In all, the fruit appears 11 times throughout the Bible.

Punica gratum takes its name from the Latin "grained apple." In its casing, the fruit can hide many hundreds of seeds. These seeds were a delicacy to the ancient Egyptians who would order them in continual supply for the Royal households.

They were a fruit useful for other purposes, too. The crimson blossom would be crushed and used as red dye. When squeezed, the peel helped to turn Moroccan leather yellow. Rich in precious moisture, the Israelites would make spiced wines from their juices. Carved Pomegranates covered the magnificent pillars of King Solomon's Temple.

They are one of the earliest cultivated fruits on record. They appear not only in the Old Testament writings but also the Qu'aran, the Homeric Hymns and ancient records from Mesopotamia. Carbonized exocarps have been found in Jericho dating right back to the early Bronze Age, approximately 3000 B.C.

Pomegranates had been cultivated in ancient Egypt for many hundreds of years by the time of the Exodus. It is thought they may have been introduced from Persia or modern-day Iran by Tutmoses III. The Ebers Papyrus records the roots of the tree were steeped as a remedy to treat roundworm.

In the Roman world, should you happen to see a woman wearing a headdress made of Pomegranate twigs, you would know she was a married lady. By A.D. 1500, Christianity had taken on the Pomegranate as a symbol of Christ's resurrection. The symbolism was a protracted version taken from the early beginnings of a Greek myth of Persephone's descent into the underworld. She was bound there to ferry the souls of the dead by Hades (through having eaten six seeds of the fruit) and only allowed to return back to the earth for half of the year. On her return, spring would come back to the world. Thus, this connection between the seeds and rebirth created a whole new symbolism for the church.

BIBLICAL REFERENCES TO POMEGRANATE

Exodus 28:34
Exodus 39:26
1 Samuel 14:2
Song of Solomon 4:3
Song of Solomon 6:7
Song of Solomon 8:2
Joel 1:12
Haggai 2:19

POMEGRANATE'S HEALING PROPERTIES

Pomegranate Seed oil is highly sought after for beauty and skin care products. Rich in phytosterols, it is considered a treasure trove of beneficial properties for the skin because of its antioxidants and punicic and egallic acids. Punicic acid is an oil known as "Super CLA," or linoleic acid, that is found to support healthy fat metabolism and weight loss. This carrier oil is an excellent base for all types of skin conditions, including eczema, sunburn, dry and cracked skin and mature skin. Pomegranate Seed oil also revives the skin's elastic nature. Research has shown the oil to actually stimulate keratinocyte production, strengthening the dermis. The oil is rich in phytoestrogens as well, which helps women manage menopause symptoms. Pomegranate Seed oil can be used alone or combined with a lotion or base oil such as Jojoba, Almond or Olive and then applied to the skin.

TRADITIONAL USES

Pomegranate Seed carrier oil is suitable for applications in both soap and skin care. It is often viewed as a facial oil in that it moisturizes and nourishes dry skin. It also balances pH, and after application, the skin usually feels soft and smooth.

MEDICINAL USES

Pomegranate absorbs into skin fairly well, with a slight oily feel though only small amounts are normally used in concert with other oils. It is considered non-toxic and non-irritant, and may be used by anyone.

Newsweek magazine reported that the Pomegranate fruit has protective benefits against cancer, heart disease, and high blood pressure. Its seeds and surrounding pulp are packed with nutrients like vitamin C and potassium. Pomegranate fruit is high in antioxidants and is helpful to prevent heart disease and stroke. Pomegranate extract is known for its amazing skin care benefits.

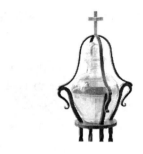

Rose of Isaiah

The Rose of Isaiah has captured the imaginations for generations. What did this flower look like? In fact, the flower does not appear to be mentioned anywhere else in the Bible except in the book of Isaiah. This may be because scholars do not believe it to be a rose as we would recognize it.

The original Hebrew word is *ha'bezzeleth*, which translates to rose or crocus. Its Semitic studies have exposed the translation to actually mean a plant with a bulb-like root. Not a rose, then – scholars agree the Rose of Isaiah is, in fact, a daffodil.

Consider the hymn "Jesus, Rose of Sharon." Strangely, no such reference appears in the Bible in relation to Christ. But in Song of Solomon 2:1, Solomon's Shulamite bride refers to herself as the Rose of Sharon. The Hebrew word Sharon (or Saron) means a level place or a plain. On the Sharon grow wild *Narcissus tazetta*, rock rose, and cistus. While the rock rose and cistus have the appearance of a rose, Narcissus is closer to the literal interpretation.

Narcissus tazetta is sometimes called "minnow" since it is a very small flower. Growing to around 18 inches, most of that is long, willowing stem. The cream-colored outer petals circle the bright yellow trumpet into a flower, which measures about 6 inches.

The original translation of Rose is the name *Habazilith*. Its root is from the same Hebrew stem word is *ha'bezzeleth*, meaning "she is peeling." Consider the layers of a woman, layer upon layer – indeed, think of *Salomes' Dance of the Seven Veils*. Furthermore, in this stem we have the layers of Heaven, Earth, and the Underworld. In modern-day language, we call this daffodil the lent lily. Think of the correlation between that of Eastern religions, which use the water lily opening to portray the opening up of enlightenment.

By saying she is peeling, Solomon's bride exposes herself as "the Layered One," which is synonymous with Bazlith, a pagan goddess of the time. *Bazlith* again comes from the stem word *bazal*, meaning onion. The daughters of Bazlith were temple servants of the time. They were, however, not attributed to Yahweh's temple, but Solomon's temple to Ashtoret, the Mother Goddess.

Israel's incomplete conquest of Canaan had meant they had not been able to vanquish the temples of Baal and the idolatry that was always a thorn in Israel's side. Ashtoret, better known by the name Astarte, or the Assyrian name Ishtar, continued to have a devout following. Solomon himself lapsed from devotion to the Lord and had a temple erected to her.

Consider the power, then, of this woman who called herself Daffodil. She had a foot in both camps, Yahweh's following and that of Ashtoret. Does her song signify the beginning of the end for the Israelite nation? Revisit Isaiah again with these thoughts in mind and you may see the rose actually is portrayed quite wantonly, very much as we would imagine exotic dancers, in fact.

Narcissus' unpleasant connotations are seeped through ancient legend and history. The Greeks of old told a tale of the son of the river god Ciphissus and the wood nymph Liorope. Narcissus was a proud man, who stood in rebuke of anyone who fell in love with him. Nemesis saw this and lured him to see his own reflection in a lake, where he instantly fell in love with his own image.

Here we have a correlation again, of seeing what is beneath the surface, peeling back the layers to understand what is happening in the layers of ourselves below. Hades pushed a daffodil up through the earth the tempt Persephone into the underworld. Even today the daffodils hang their heads in shame for the part they played in her abduction and in mourning for her mother Demeter who was left behind.

The low germination point of the daffodil makes it a very toxic plant, and as one would guess, it is neurotoxic. The Shamans use its hallucinogenic properties to show a person what lies beneath. What's interesting to note in revisiting Persephone's myth, is that only when we are stripped to the core during times of hardship do we truly find out who we are and what we are capable of. One has to wonder what might be the symbolism, then, behind the discovery of a *Narcissus tazetta* bulb in the neck of the mummy of Ramses II.

BIBLICAL REFERENCES TO ROSE OF ISAIAH

Isaiah 35:1

ROSE OF ISAIAH'S HEALING PROPERTIES

As part of the daffodil family, the Rose of Isaiah mentioned in the Bible is not actually a rose plant. The Narcissus genus is spread across Europe, Africa, and Asia, with over 50 recognized species.

Narcissus plants belong to the Amaryllidaceae family. This species, the *Narcissus tazetta*, is native to the Holy Land and grows on the Plain of Sharon in Israel. The essential oil is produced from its distinctively shaped flowers by a process of enfleurage or solvent extraction. It has a sweet, floral, and fruity scent that blends well with Rose, Sandalwood, Jasmine, Neroli, Ylang Ylang and other floral oils.

Interestingly, *Narcissus tazetta* contains a subtle, unique fragrance – also found in roses – which is recognized by bees, but almost unperceivable to the human nose.

TRADITIONAL USES

Narcissus tazetta was first used to treat tumors in ancient Chinese medicine, as its bulbs contain pretazettine, a naturally occurring antitumor chemical. Evidence of the plant was also discovered in ancient Egyptian tombs.

The plant has a long history of its use as a stimulant and was used by ancient Romans to treat abscesses, wounds, and muscular pains. Its flowers were crushed into a syrup and prescribed as a remedy for dysentery. Across Europe, Narcissus flowers were used as an antispasmodic, aphrodisiac, contraceptive and even a cure for baldness.

Narcissus tazetta is believed to be the 'desert rose' that is mentioned in the Book of Isaiah. It is sometimes referred to as the Rose of Sharon, on account of its natural habitation on the Plain of Sharon.

MEDICINAL USES

Although not used in modern aromatherapy, Rose of Isaiah has been used to treat tumors, bacterial infections, headaches, epilepsy, hysteria, skin infections, and stress-related disorders.

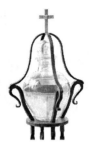

Rose of Sharon

In ancient times, the *Cistus ladanifer,* also known as the "rock rose," was believed to be the Rose of Sharon. As goats and sheep roamed through the brush, this flower became entangled in their coats. While caring for their sheep, the shepherds would collect it from their wool and rub the resin on their cuts and wounds to soothe them.

This multi-petal flower is found in the fertile plain called Sharon between Jaffa and Mount Carmel in Israel. Rose of Sharon has a honey scent from an aromatic gum that exudes from the plant.

The Hebrew word *sharon* (Strong's #2261) means "meadow-saffron, crocus, and rose (place of pasture)." It is a derivative for Sarai, which means "princess."

Think of how the thornless Rose of Sharon beautifully mirrors Yeshua's tender love, as spoken of in Song of Solomon 2:1: *I am the rose of Sharon and the lily of the valleys.* The Scriptures tell believers that they are the sheep of his pasture and feed among the lilies.

BIBLICAL REFERENCES TO ROSE OF SHARON

Song of Solomon 2:1

ROSE OF SHARON'S HEALING PROPERTIES

Rose of Sharon essential oil a sticky brown resin obtained from the shrubs of the *Cistus ladanifer* species. It has a long history of use in herbal medicine and as a perfume ingredient. Labdanum is a small, sticky shrub that grows up to 3 meters high with fragrant white flowers and lance-shaped leaves that are white and furry on the underside. This multi-petal flower is found in the fertile plain called Sharon between Jaffa and Mount Carmel in Israel. It has a honey scent from an aromatic gum that exudes from the plant.

TRADITIONAL USES

In biblical times, shepherds would use Rose of Sharon resin to heal cuts and wounds. Their goats and sheep would roam around and collect the flowers on their woolen coats, allowing the shepherds to benefit from this natural remedy. The essential oil was also traditionally used as an anti-inflammatory and remedy to stop bleeding. With a spiritual connection, cistus essential oil has been used for meditation since ancient times. It is believed to open the 'third eye' chakra and induce calmness.

MEDICINAL USES

Rose of Sharon has been studied for its therapeutic effect on cell regeneration according to Dr. David Stewart, author of *Healing Oils of the Bible*.

Rose of Sharon has been used for bronchitis, respiratory infections, urinary tract infections, wounds, and wrinkles. It is also known to be anti-infectious, antiviral, and antibacterial. Rose of Sharon helps to reduce inflammation and acts as a powerful antihemorrhaging agent. The *Essential Oils Desk Reference, 5th Edition* reports that it also helps strengthen the immune system. Rose of Sharon helps to quiet the nerves and elevate the emotions during prayer. Studies revealed that people taking antidepressant drugs found this oil to be mood-elevating by rubbing it on their bodies or just inhaling it.

Its infection-fighting properties make it a good oil for treating respiratory conditions, such as bronchitis, colds, coughs and rhinitis. *Cistus ladanifer* can also be used to treat urinary tract infections. As a neurotonic, it supports the sympathetic nervous system and boosts immunity. Its ability to stimulate cell regeneration means Cistus labdanum oil can be used as a skin treatment for wrinkles, aging skin, cuts and wounds. It helps to reduce hemorrhage and inflammation, which can bring relief to arthritic aches and pains. Emotionally, its relaxing scent can help to lift the spirits and calm the nerves.

SPICE CHEST: THE SENSE OF SMELL

Smelling the fragrance of a rose can bring healing and elevate one's mood. Even when the scent is too faint to notice healing is taking place. The sense of smell facilitated through the olfactory nerve invites the fragrance into certain regions of the brain, enabling the body to process them naturally.

Just inhaling a fragrance will bring healing to the body because with pure therapeutic essential oils the molecules are small enough to bypass the blood-brain barrier and reach down at the cellular level to bring. Regular inhalation of essential oils stimulates the limbic region of the brain and encourages the natural release of the human growth hormone or HGH.

With 1,000 sensors in the nose, it can identify 10,000 scents. And because the nose is wired differently that the other four senses, it carries molecules directly into the emotional center of the brain where traumatic memories are stored. Essential oils are a vehicle by which repressed emotions can be release.

The Hebrew word for "smell" is *reyach*, and this shares the same root word for "spirit," which is *ruach*. Yahweh was moved to compassion by the sense of smell as in the account of Noah's offering after the flood: *And Noah builded an altar unto the LORD... and offered burnt offerings... and the LORD smelled a sweet savour; and the LORD said in his heart, I will not again curse the ground any more for man's sake* (Genesis 8:20-21).

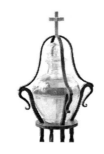

Rue

Ruta graveolens is cited on one occasion in the Bible in Luke 11:42.

> *Woe to you Pharisees, because you give God a tenth of your Mint, Rue and all other kinds of garden herbs, but you neglect justice and the love of God. You should have practiced the latter without leaving the former undone.*

Notice the similarity in tone to Matthew 23:23, and while it seems to speak of the same instance in history, Rue does not appear in the passage in Matthew.

We know Rue was one of the herbs to be tithed to the temple, and again Jesus accuses the Pharisees of not being true in their commitment to the Lord. Here, though, he is precise, because a new commitment to God is called for, but they still must continue to tithe the herbs. This greater interest in the weightier issues of love and compassion are on top of the tithe to the temple. As yet, then, the new commandments of God are not seen as coming back into play. At this point in history, a person was expected to tithe amounts as much as 23% of their income. Later, we read of a new commitment to give as much as you can afford. Herbs, of course, are an easier tender than that of entirety of heart to God's work.

Rue grew very easily in Israel. It is a small shrub with lovely yellow flowers with an unyielding odor. As early as the 2nd century A.D., records from the ancient Greek gynecologist Soranus describe Rue as an abortifacient. Indeed today, aromatherapists avoid use of this essential oil as it impedes blood flow to the endometrium.

The tithe of Rue suggests it would have had use in the temple, and throughout history it has been used as an antibacterial. Most notably it is a component of the four thieves' vinegar. While the origins of the vinegar are unknown, one story suggests it was made by a family of perfumers to hide their scent as they stole from houses during the plague. Another attributes it to robbers who were condemned to the corpses in the plague of 18th century France. Or, perhaps it originated in New Orleans to prevent the bites of malaria.

The common thread running through is its dispersal of insects. In the Middle Ages, Rue leaves were swept through the house to dispel fleas, which could have carried the plague from rats.

The Romans attributed Rue to their god Mars and would plant it around the outside of their temples. It is also attributed to Diane and Arcadia. They used Rue to consecrate items made of iron, interestingly also attributed to Mars.

Rue was known to define a warrior. Its blue feathery leaves irritated the skin of those who were sensitive. A person who could tolerate Rue was a fighter indeed.

Early Christians referred to Rue as the herb of grace, using it as part of their ritual exorcisms and masses, while aspersing with holy water to sanctify a soul. It is said the Prophet Mohammed blessed his followers with it as well.

Rue has been used since Roman times to sooth strained eyes and over the centuries became endowed with the power to bring second sight.

In medieval times, Rue was carried by people to ward off witches, and if they saw an enemy they might throw the herb at them as a curse. This is the origin of the saying, "You'll rue the day."

BIBLICAL REFERENCES TO RUE

Luke 11:42

RUE'S HEALING PROPERTIES

Rue is an herb, sometimes known as herb-of-grace, which is native to the Balkan Peninsula of Europe. The plant belongs to the Rutaceae family and has been used for medicinal and culinary purposes since biblical times. It is no longer commonly used in modern aromatherapy.

By steam distilling the leaves of the plant, an essential oil is produced that is normally solid at room temperature. Rue has a sharp, fruity, herbaceous scent that blends well with Chamomile, Myrrh, Bay, Fennel, Frankincense, Thyme and Benzoin, among others.

TRADITIONAL USES

Rue was used by the ancient Greeks to protect against witchcraft, which was a theory that continued well into the Middle Ages. The herb featured in a medieval wellness guide, which described the ability of Rue to "sharpen the eyesight and dissipate flatulence". As well as improving regular eyesight, herbalists believed Rue had the ability to provide second sight. It was also widely believed to act as an antidote to poison.

Rue was used to encourage the onset of menstruation and stimulate uterine contractions, therefore acting as an abortifacient. Other traditional uses for Rue included remedies for epilepsy, sciatica and vertigo.

Court judges would often be presented with bouquets of Rue to ward off fleas and pests that may have been transferred into court from prisoners. In Lithuania, it was traditional for virgin brides to wear Rue at their wedding, to symbolize purity.

As its name suggests, Rue symbolizes regret in many famous literary works, such as *Paradise Lost* and *Gulliver's Travels*. It was one of the flowers scattered by Ophelia in Shakespeare's "Hamlet." The herb is also mentioned in the Bible as one of the tithed goods.

MEDICINAL USES

Rue was traditionally used to treat nervous disorders, such as convulsions, as well as menstrual problems, arthritis, stress and insomnia. Its antiseptic qualities made it a popular skin treatment for bacterial and fungal infections, bites and stings. It was also a common digestive remedy for food poisoning, colic, loss of appetite and indigestion.

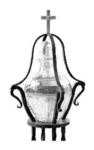

Saffron

Crocus sativus or Saffron is known as one of the most expensive spices and has herbaceous, warm, woodsy aroma. Saffron comes from an orange-yellow flower of the Crocus family. Saffron is literally worth its weight in gold because it is the stigmas from which the spice is obtained. Each one is handpicked and placed over a charcoal fire for drying. It takes over 75,000 flowers to make one pound of Saffron. One of the earliest historical references mentioning Saffron comes out of ancient Egypt where the stigmas were used in perfumes, as a drug, for hair and fabric dye, as well as for culinary purposes.

Saffron was used by Cleopatra as an aromatic and seductive essence, and to make ablutions in temples. Crocus flowers, from which Saffron is obtained, were considered sacred in Crete. It was regarded as a ancient symbol of the sun and was used to dye foods the color yellow as part of solar worship.

Saffron was strewn in Greek halls, courts, theaters, and baths as perfume. In Rome, Saffron was sprinkled in the streets when Nero made his entry into the city. In Rome, the Roman emperors were famous for their extravagance, which included spraying Saffron from fountains and using it as a strewing herb.

During the Renaissance, it was worth its weight in gold and today is still the most expensive spice in the world. Its high price led to its adulteration, which was severely punished by Henry VIII, even including condemning to death adulterers of Saffron.

The only verse in the scriptures that mentions Saffron is in the Song of Solomon. Song of Solomon 4:14 says,

> *Spikenard and saffron, calamus and Cinnamon, with all trees of Frankincense; Myrrh and Aloes, with all the chief spices.*

Spiritually, Saffron symbolizes the costly but triumphant faith of the Messiah against his enemy. Now believers can live by faith, just as the disciples did, knowing that the testing of their faith through fire will be more precious than gold. 1 Peter 1:7-8 says,

That the trial of your faith, being much more precious than of gold that perisheth, though it be tried with fire, might be found unto praise and honour and glory at the appearing of Yeshua Ha Machiach: Whom having not seen, ye love; in whom, though now ye see him not, yet believing, ye rejoice with joy unspeakable and full of glory.

Hebrews 11:6 tells us:

But without faith it is impossible to please him: for he that cometh to God must believe that he is and that he is a rewarder of them that diligently seek him.

Allow the Lord to complete his perfect work in your character and place these beautiful fragrances in the garden of your heart.

The Hebrew word for Saffron (Strong's #3750) is *karkom*, which identifies it as an orange-yellow flower of the crocus family, which is used for flavoring in drinks and confections in order to promote perspiration for cooling of the body.

BIBLICAL REFERENCES TO SAFFRON

Song of Solomon 4:14

SAFFRON'S HEALING PROPERTIES

Saffron is loaded with natural compounds that have potential health benefits and, therefore, is widely used as an ingredient in both western and eastern medicine to treat several diseases and disorders. It is said to have active ingredients that lower blood pressure. It also has compounds that increase antibacterial and antiviral physiological activity in the body. The presence of crocetin makes it helpful in reducing the blood cholesterol levels and triglycerides and strengthening the heart and nervous system. Researches have demonstrated the memory-enhancing, anti-cancer and antioxidant activities of Saffron extracts.

TRADITIONAL USES

Folkloric uses of Saffron have included its use as a sedative, expectorant, aphrodisiac and diaphoretic. It is said to be beneficial in curing conditions like sore gums, heart and lung disease, common colds, kidney stones, alcoholism, cramps, insomnia, menstrual problems, diabetes, asthma, and depression. It is also known to have anti-aging properties and is used in skin lightening and anti-aging creams and other beauty products. It is also is a potent antioxidant that relieves both pain and inflammation. A few drops of Saffron essential oil may be mixed with half a teaspoon of Almond oil and rubbed directly into the joints for this purpose. Saffron is said to help in digestion and increases appetite. It is also used to get relief from renal colic and stomach aches.

MEDICINAL USES

Saffron has many medicinal uses. A 2010 double-blind, placebo-controlled study found Saffron helped mild to moderate Alzheimer's disease. Crocetin, an important carotenoid constituent of Saffron, has shown significant potential as an anti-tumor agent in animal models and cell culture systems. Saffron inhibits DMBA-induced skin carcinoma in mice when treated early. Both Saffron stigma and petals are said to be helpful for depression. Satiereal (Inoreal Ltd, Plerin, France), a novel extract of Saffron stigma, may reduce snacking and enhance satiety through its suggested mood-improving effect, and thus contribute to weight loss. Saffron was found to be effective in relieving symptoms of PMS. Saffron, crocins, and crocetin inhibit breast cancer cell proliferation. Crocus sativus (most Saffron research refers to the stigmas but often this is not made clear in research papers) inhibits histamine H1 receptors in animals, suggesting a potential use in allergic disorders. Histamine is a biological amine that plays a significant role in allergic responses. Saffron may have a protective effect on the heart.

A recent (2011) double-blind human trial found use of 100 mg of Saffron daily has temporary immunomodulatory activities.

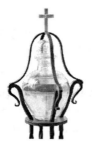

Sandalwood

Santalum album is a highly prized aromatic wood that is grown primarily in India. Its wood is used for making furniture, ornaments, sacred objects, carvings and incense while its essential oil is used in medicine, perfume, and aromatherapy. There are sixteen species of Sandalwood grown naturally throughout the Pacific and Eastern Indian Ocean regions. Historical records indicate that the Sandalwood tree is indigenous to mountain districts of south India and Malayan Archipelago. Plant biologists describe the tree as indigenous to Southeast Asia, and say it was introduced to India by traders. Today, almost 90% of the world's population of Sandalwood oil is from India.

As an evergreen, it ranges in size from tall scrubs to tall trees. Sandalwood is a parasitic plant, which means its root structure has the ability to penetrate the roots of host plants to obtain nutrients. One of the most famous varieties, *Mysore* Sandalwood from India, has been reduced greatly to the point of extinction and is now protected as an endangered species from harvesting.

Aura Cacia's website reports:

"Trees harvested for oil are selected by age and size because of the higher proportion of heartwood (and thus essential oil) in larger trees. Dead-standing or fallen trees are also harvested because the wood holds onto the essential oil for many years. The whole tree is harvested and used – including the sawdust and the stump (which has the highest oil content) and the sapwood (which contains a small amount of oil). The lower grades of Sandalwood, such as the sapwood, are used for incense and for chips and powder while the better logs are used in carving (from small objects to furniture)."

Today, Sandalwood is used for intricate carvings, furniture, and various ornaments. Chips of wood are burned as an incense or ground to make incense sticks.

Sandalwood was first used over 4,000 years ago in Egypt, Greece, and Rome. It has been valued as one of the most sacred trees as an important part of devotional rituals. In India, the Sandalwood has been used to make various religious artifacts such as staffs and figurines, and deities of different kinds which were installed in a shrine or temple or placed upon the home altar. Chips of wood are burned as an incense in temples or on personal altars as a reminder of the fragrant realms of the heavens.

As an important medicinal herb, Sandalwood was used in traditional Chinese and Tibetan medicines and in Indian healing science known as Ayurveda. Historical records indicate that by 700 B.C., it had been found in Egyptian embalming formulas as well as other culture's death rituals such as India's custom of burning on funeral pyres or using its wood for making coffins for the very wealthy. Many temples and structures were built from Sandalwood.

For more than 2,000 years, Sandalwood has been a favorite ingredient in perfumes, incense, lotions and body oils. In China, Sandalwood is very popular for joss sticks as incense. Sandalwood's popularity in the European and American perfumery was not significant until the 1900s, where it was appreciated for its fixative ability as well as its amazing fragrance. To this day, it is still often used in fine perfumes.

In the Hebrew, Sandalwood is translated *almug* and occurs four times in scripture.

BIBLICAL REFERENCES TO SANDALWOOD

1 Kings 10:11
1 Kings 10:12
11 Chronicles 2:8
11 Chronicles 9:10-11

SANDALWOOD'S HEALING PROPERTIES

Sandalwood is an evergreen tree that comes from the Sandalwood family. Growing from 16 species in Asia, Australia, and on the islands in the Pacific Ocean, Sandalwood grows mostly in sandy areas with rocky soil and dry conditions, in deciduous forests, and can be found in deserts, valleys, and mountains about 8,000 feet above sea level.

Sandalwood's soft and rich balsamic odor falls in the classic oriental woody base note category with a delightful lingering scent. Its sweet fragrance lasts a long time and has been used in all types of perfume compositions, especially Indian attars.

The Sandalwood tree takes a very long time to grow and produces the best oil by around 80 years old, but oil can be extracted when the tree is 40 years old. The tree can reach anywhere from 33 to 66 feet in height and is known to be semi-parasite, which means it can survive on its own without the need for other plants or insects.

In India, Sandalwood is considered beneficial for meditation and for calming and quieting the mind. Drops of Sandalwood essential oil can be applied to the forehead, the temples, or rubbed between the eyebrows before prayer or meditation. It is believed to help to set the mood and prepare the mind to begin its inward journey.

TRADITIONAL USES

Sandalwood has been known to have the properties of antispasmodic (relieving spasms of the muscles), antibacterial and antiviral. It is also used in the treatment of fever, flu, heart and stomach issues, skin disorders, gums of the teeth, and rashes.

For a long time, Sandalwood was used in many civilizations and religions of the world. In Hinduism, it was considered holy and indispensable in all of the social and religious rituals. Ranging from a person's birth until their death, Sandalwood played a significant part. It was presented as an offering to their gods, used as a decorative item for a baby's birthday, used for embalming a family member's body at burial, and worn on a person's forehead, which is very common in India.

MEDICINAL USES

Sandalwood is very effective towards inflammation of all types like in the brain, digestive, and nervous systems. It has a cooling effect and can provide relief from burns and can also help quickly heal old wounds such as scars. It is known to help combat side effects of antibiotics, poisoning, and insect bites or wounds. Sandalwood has both relaxant and sedative properties, which can help ease muscle spasms.

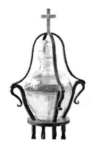

Spikenard

There are three accounts in the Scriptures of Yeshua being anointed with Spikenard, found in Luke 7:36-38, Mark 14:3 and John 12:1-3.

This rare and costly fragrant oil was used by Mary of Bethany to anoint the head and feet of the Messiah two days before his death, as recorded in the Gospel of John. The amount of Spikenard essential oil that was poured on Jesus, one alabaster box of Spikenard, would have cost a common laborer at the time of our Savior a year's worth of wages.

Pure Spikenard is a very costly spice called "nard," in the King James Version, which comes from the Hebrew word *nard* meaning "light." Interestingly, the message delivered in 1 John 1:5 talked about the nature of the Father, who is visible in Heaven by the pure, created light of his nature. Yeshua himself shared in this glory at the Mount of Transfiguration when the divine light was visible as he transfigured in a whiteness that was beyond any earthly whiteness as described in Mark 9:3.

Soon, his bride will share in this glorious apparel as our wedding apparel, mentioned in the book of Revelation. Revelation 19:8 says,

> *And to her was granted that she should be arrayed in fine linen, clean and white; for the fine linen is the righteousness of saints.*

In the Old Testament in the Song of Solomon 1:12 it says,

> *While the king sitteth at his table, my Spikenard sendeth forth the smell thereof.*

In this verse, the King is sitting, symbolic of his finished work at Calvary's tree. He invites his Bride to come and join him for a marriage supper feast at his table. Here is pictured the Bride and her fragrance that emanates out of her spirit in worship and adoration for the King's provision – a heavenly fragrance all should possess.

Solomon's prophecy was fulfilled a thousand years later in John 12:3, where the Bible tells how Spikenard was used to anoint Yeshua, the pure and spotless Lamb, just days before his death and burial.

Then Mary took a pound of ointment of Spikenard, very costly, and anointed the feet of Jesus, and wiped his feet with her hair, and the house was filled with the odor of the ointment.

Mark 14:3 tells us of another woman who came having an alabaster flask of very precious oil of Spikenard, and she broke the seal and poured the oil on Yeshua's head. Some of the disciples were very indignant with the "waste" of costly oil, as it may have cost this woman as much as a whole year's wages. But Yeshua rebuked them and said she had done a good work, preparing him for his death, for her deed would be remembered wherever the gospel would be preached.

The Greek word for Spikenard is *nardos*, meaning "genuine or pure."

Those desiring to become the spotless Bride of Messiah must walk in purity and light, with a pure, genuine heart of devotion. With his life broken, he doesn't leave believers alone to "waste away." Instead, the oil, symbolic of the inner working of the Ruach HaKodesh (Holy Spirit), has been poured out, so believers can live a life that is rich with a sweet, heavenly fragrane.

SPICE CHEST: SPIKENARD – A FRAGRANCE SENT FORTH!

While the king sitteth at his table, my Spikenard sendeth forth the smell thereof. Song of Solomon 1:12.

The exotic smell of Spikenard is introduced again in the Song of Solomon 1:12. In C.R. Oliver's book, *Solomon's Secret,* the author describes how the Shulamite's fragrant Spikenard wafts the Shepherd-King with her deep adoration, love, and devotion to him. Interestingly, she chooses the word "sendeth," Oliver explains. Like a scriptural flag for the reader to take notice of, she describes this costly ointment as being "sent forth" just as Yeshua's disciples were "sent out." Oliver says:

"The Bible says the word of God is 'sent forth' to heal. A specific reason, task, or design is associated with the action of this verb. It is one thing to have an exotic perfume present, but to send it forth as if to accomplish a specific purpose is something else. Ointment in the Song is sent forth to herald another event which had not yet taken place, an event of history which even His disciples could not fathom."

We see Solomon's prophecy fulfilled in the New Testament, in the account of the woman with the alabaster box who anointed the Lord before his death and burial. The disciples considered her action a "waste," but Yeshua said her gift of anointing was a good deed and would be remembered wherever the gospel was preached.

As a prophetic fulfillment, blending these fragrant accounts of Scripture together connects time and history for us. Solomon places the ointment of Spikenard in opening act of the Song of Songs as a reminder to the fragrant mixture that perfumed the door of the tabernacle during the worship services. He wanted to make sure there is no mistake of who he was writing about – our High Priest and King, Yeshua!

BIBLICAL REFERENCES TO SPIKENARD

Song of Solomon 1:2
Song of Solomon 4:13
Song of Solomon 4:14
Matthew 26:7
Mark 14:3
Luke 7:37
John 12:3

SPIKENARD'S HEALING PROPERTIES

Spikenard or *Nardostachys jatamansi* is also commonly known as false Indian Valerian Root essential oil. Nard is taken from the root of the plant and has a strong, earthy aromatic odor. It was prized in early Egypt as one of the early aromatics produced by the Egyptians and mentioned frequently throughout ancient writings. It was also popular in the Middle East during the time of our Savior.

Spikenard essential oil is 93% sesquiterpenes, which have the ability to oxygenate the brain. Spikenard comes from a very rare plant that is usually blended with Olive oil for anointing acts of consecration, dedication, and worship.

TRADITIONAL USES

Spikenard essential oil is highly regarded in India as a perfume, medicinal herb, and skin tonic. In ancient times, it was the one of the most precious oils used only by priests, kings, or high initiates. References in the New Testament describe how Mary of Bethany used a salve of Spikenard to anoint the feet of Jesus before the Passover.

MEDICINAL USES

Spikenard is helpful in the treatment of allergic skin reactions and skin cancer. It may also help with allergies, Candida, indigestion, insomnia, menstrual difficulties, migraines, nausea, rashes, bacterial infections, stress, tachycardia, tension, and wounds that will not heal. According to Dietrich Gumbel, Ph.D. it strengthens the heart and circulatory system. It is very relaxing and acts as a natural sedaive.

Spikenard is known to be antibacterial, antifungal, anti-inflammatory, a deodorant, and a skin tonic. It is 93% sesquiterpenes in content and can erase incorrect information in the DNA or cellular memory.

SPICE CHEST: ANOINTING OF THE FEET

In biblical times, it was customary for visitors traveling long distances over dusty roads to be welcomed warmly with a foot washing followed by anointing with oil as an expression of Jewish hospitality. This is mentioned in Genesis 18:4 and Genesis 24:32.

In the New Testament, Yeshua made mention of this custom when he was invited to a Pharisee's house for dinner, and they did not extend this act of hospitality to him.

In the gospel of Luke, Yeshua was anointed by an uninvited woman at the gathering where she washed his feet with her tears and then wiped them with her hair. In Luke 7:36-38, it says:

> And one of the Pharisees desired him
> that he would eat with him. And he
> went into the Pharisee's house and sat
> down to meat. And, behold, a woman
> in the city, which was a sinner, when
> she knew that Jesus sat at meat in

the Pharisee's house, brought an alabaster box of ointment, and stood at his feet behind him weeping, and begun to wash his feet with tears, and did wipe them with the hairs of her head, and kissed his feet, and anointed them with the ointment.

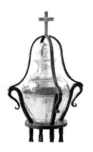

Terebinth

Terebinth appears many times throughout the Old Testament and on most occasions the term comes under scrutiny with its close translation to that of Oak. Its many forms are *Elah*, *El* (but only ever used in its plural *elim*) *Elon*, *allah* and *allon*. All of these are interchangeable between the species.

What makes this even more complicated is the outward appearance of the trees is also very similar. They are deciduous and have widely spread, majestic-looking branches. Both oaks and Terebinth, *Pisticia terebinthus*, were used as favorite sites of religious practice, not least because of the frequencies of theophanies at these tress. The appearances of deities to humans or other beings appear with regularity in the Old Testament; for example, in Genesis 18:1, when the Lord appears to Abraham:

> *And the LORD appeared unto him among the terebinth trees of Mamre, and he was sitting in the door of his tent in the heat of the day.*

These sightings made the grounds of the Terebinth to be hallowed ground. The description of Deborah's burial under the tree in Genesis 38:8 seems to be unanimously ascribed to the Oak despite it having the same translated name. It should, of course, be noted their sheer presence of appearance and longevity in one place might just as likely have made them chosen as landmarks easy to spot.

> *Now Deborah, Rebekah's nurse, died and was buried under the oak outside Bethel. So it was named Allon Bakuth.*

In Isaiah 44:14, we discover the folly of idolatry. Some translations lead us to believe idols were made from Terebinth; others see it more that people were actually worshipping the trees. It seems likely that the former be most accurate; however, because of their robust nature both tress came to be symbols of strength and longevity.

Pisticia terebinthus is a shrub native to the Canary Islands but grew throughout the Mediterranean. This is more commonly known not only as Terebinth but also the turpentine tree and is the shrub we would associate as Terebinth today. (This was one of the earliest sources of resin for turpentine). In Palestine grows various species, which also grew right through the Levant in biblical times. This was *Pisticia palestina*. Its egg-shaped leaves sit on wider spreading branches than its more common Terebinth cousin.

BIBLICAL REFERENCES TO TEREBINTH

Genesis 35:4
Judges 6:11
Judges 6:19
Joshua 24:26
2 Samuel 18:9
2 Samuel 18:10
2 Samuel 18:14
1 Kings 13:14
1 Chronicles 10:12
Isaiah 1:30
Isaiah 6:13
Ezekiel 6:13

TEREBINTH'S HEALING PROPERTIES

A close relative of the pistachio, the *Pistacia terebinthus* plant produces Terebinth resin, one of the earliest sources of turpentine. Unlike common turpentine, which is produced by Pine trees, Terebinth is from the Anacardiaceae family. Native to the Mediterranean region, it is also known as Indian Turpentine or turpentine tree.

Terebinth essential oil is extracted by hydro-distillation of its aerial parts. The clear oil has a warm, balsamic scent that blends well with Benzoin, Cypress, and Eucalyptus.

TRADITIONAL USES

Terebinth was used for aromatic and medicinal purposes in classical Greece. The Terebinth tree is referenced in the Bible when the Angel of the Lord appeared to Gideon. The Angel helped Gideon to realize his inner strength and gave him the courage he needed to fulfill his call to God's service. It symbolizes strength and resistance, as the tree grows in mountainous areas where other plants fail to survive. In Hebrew, the tree is called *Elah*, which means "God the strong one."

MEDICINAL USES

Although not commonly used in modern aromatherapy, Terebinth can be used to treat digestive disorders, urinary infections, muscular aches and pains, respiratory problems and skin conditions. It can also boost poor circulation and soothe neuralgia and sciatica.

In traditional Iranian medicine, *Pistacia terebinthus* was used as an aphrodisiac and remedy for liver, heart, kidney and respiratory disorders. The resin was traditionally used internally to treat bronchial infections, urinary infections, hemorrhages, gallstones, and rheumatism. Externally, Terebinth was applied in the form of liniments, enemas, and baths, for everything from digestive problems, menstrual disorders, arthritis, burns and respiratory conditions.

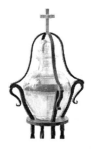

Wormwood

Wormwood, the herb that was later to become the legendary drink first made by French witches called absinthe, is used in the Bible to depict bitterness. It is easy to see why the symbolism was chosen as it does indeed taste very sour. Proverbs 5:4 reads,

> *...but in the end she is bitter as wormwood,*
> *sharp as a two-edged sword.*

Artemisia of many varieties grew throughout Palestine. It is mentioned several times throughout the Old Testament but its most famous mention is in the book of Revelation. Many theologians suspect the translation *apsinthos* means "star or angel" and pinpointed a rising political figure for that time. Is it a prophecy of the future or it is communicating events of that period? Most likely it pertains to a leader of persecution of some sort, a governor or even a description of how the doctrines of the ancient church had become polluted by outside influences.

Revelation 8:10-11 says:

> *The third angel sounded his trumpet, and a great star, blazing like a torch, fell from the sky on a third of the rivers and on the springs of water – the name of the star is Wormwood. A third of the waters turned bitter, and many people died from the waters that had become bitter.*

Many have attributed this scripture to refer to the attack of the Huns lead by Atilla. A large part of their argument sings back to the earlier attribution that God would make the people drink bitter drinks from Gall plants. These drinks were made from Opium Poppy plants and Wormwood and served as a depiction of bitter punishment.

As you will see, the words differ slightly between translations. These differences in the meanings between Gall and Wormwood build the foundation for the argument for Atilla being the wormwood in the book of Revelation.

In Lamentations 3:15 (NIV) it reads, *He has filled me with bitter herbs and given me gall to drink.*

While the King James Version of Lamentations 3:15 states, *He hath filled me with bitterness, he hath made me drunken with wormwood.*

But then a few verses later in Lamentations 3:19 (KJV), it speaks of both: *Remember my affliction and my wanderings, the wormwood and the gall!*

Does that mean, then, they are not the same, and the writer actually meant to have two meanings? The same happens in Jeremiah 23:15:

> *Therefore thus saith the LORD of hosts concerning the prophets; Behold, I will feed them with wormwood, and make them drink the water of gall: for from the prophets of Jerusalem is profaneness gone forth into all the land.*

Atilla had declared war on Rome in A.D. 440 after he had failed to hold up his end of a treaty made by Theodosius. They had formerly agreed to open trade with the Huns and to pay ransom for any prisoner taken by the Hun army. Feeling they had not honored their end of the bargain, Atilla advanced on Rome and attacked at the Danube in A.D. 450.

In A.D. 451, he declared war on the Western Empire and headed towards France. (Compare Gall plants and the country of Gaul.) The Huns ransacked towns throughout their rebellion of France. Only upon encountering the Visigoths at the battle of Troyes was the rampage stilled. Later in A.D. 476, the Visigoth Odacer was to take the throne of Romulus Augustulus to become King of Italy and end the Roman Empire. He was the first barbarian ever to rule, and it marked their superiority over all of mankind. Could Wormwood be referring to the beginning of the end of the Roman Empire?

BIBLICAL REFERENCES TO WORMWOOD

Deuteronomy 29:18
Proverbs 5:4
Jeremiah 9:15
Jeremiah 23:15
Lamentations 3:15
Lamentations 3:19
Revelation 8:11

SPICE CHEST: SUN GOD WORSHIP

Perhaps Wormwood's reference in prophecy relates to the changes in the Christian doctrine bought about by the Emperor Constantine. He was the longest serving and the first Christian Roman Emperor. It is believed he converted to Christianity in A.D. 312, but evidence shows he was not actually baptized until close to the end of his life. In February A.D. 313, he legalized Christianity making it possible for the Church to practice unchallenged, and religious items that had been confiscated were returned to the Church. The previous alternative had been martyrdom. This was a huge step forward for the Church; so much so, Constantine is often referred to as *the Thirteenth Apostle*.

Documentary evidence for that time shows him taking on the symbol of the cho-rho as his emblem and moving less and less away from pagan worship, preferring to spend time in prayer with the Christians. Indeed, he attributes his rise to fame as to having Christ and God on his side.

However, despite being a converted Christian, Constantine never gave up his former devotion to the sun god, Sol Inviticus. Indeed, even the coins he had minted depicted the sun god. At his A.D. 312 triumph of the Battle of Milivian Bridge, it was marked by the construction of a celebratory arch with no Christian symbols displayed. Instead, it was covered with depictions of the goddess Victoria, with sacrifices made to Apollo, Diana, and Hercules. This victory, you will recall, was the year of his supposed conversion.

Like many pre-Christians, he continued to not only worship the Lord, but also the sun god. The writings of Clement of Alexandria depict Christ as a sun god racing his chariot across the sky. Christians met on Sunday instead of the Sabbath and by the 4th century, the birthday of the sun god was given the date of the nativity of the Christ Child.

According to the Scriptures, not all men died from the bitter waters, though. Could this possibly refer to the change in attitude of Rome towards Christianity? Under his rule, many people died for their faith in Christ, but then it stopped. Martyrdom ends when Christianity is legalized.

Historians remind us Constantine was primarily unconcerned with the theological debates of the Church. His primary concern was to bring about peace and calm within the Church. This he achieved very well, but the result may have been the Wormwood bitterness for the true Christians who resented this dilution of devotion to their one true God.

Other scholars suggest the reference might pertain to a priest from Alexandria, who served under Constantine. His theory Arianism questioned the relationship between God the Father and God the Son. His hypothesis was that because the Lord had been self-mutable and nothing had created him, meant Christ must be subordinate to him. Christ, by contrast, was a created being and so therefore was not truly divine. He, being called into being, could also then have had no prior experience of God, since God is of a different order of existence.

This theory rocked the Church and dissent was rife. Many followers were furious at this supposition that their savior was inferior, and bitterness doesn't even come close to a description. Wormwood? Quite possibly.

Or, could it be a reference to Pelagius who made radical claims against predestination by opposing the theory of Original Sin? He said, by contrast, man was free to exercise free will, to do good acts and had not been wounded by Adam's original sin in Genesis. This has interesting parallels from a passage in Brewer's dictionary, which says Wormwood was supposed to have sprung up in the track of the serpent as it writhed away from Paradise.

In his essay "Wormwood," Gerard D. Bouw asserts Wormwood's most likely meaning was of a different celestial being, that of a comet. It is true, too, that a comet or asteroid would spread a nitric acid wash that would turn the water sour.

For any readers who wonder at the imagery of a nuclear bomb, Chernobyl is also supposed to be a suggested translation of Wormwood. This is nearly true, but not quite. The name of the town is made up of two Russian stem words *chornyi* meaning black and *byllia* meaning grass blades and stalks. This pertains to a sister plant of *Artemesia absinthium*, which was grown nearby the *Artemisia vulgaris*, known as Mugwort or sometimes known as the unpalatable one. It is suggested this urban myth originates from a *New York Times* article printed on July 25, 1986, entitled, "Chernobyl Fall Out: Apocalyptic Tale." Its author Serge Schmemann attributes the incorrect translation to a "prominent Russian writer" who seems to need to remain nameless.

While most commonly attributed to *Artemesia absinthe*, the Wormwood of the Bible might also have been *Artemesia judiaca*, which grew extremely prolifically throughout Egypt. We know this less toxic strain was in common usage in the Egyptian medicinal chest. In the Papyrus Ebers in 1550 B.C., it is described as expelling worms. Soranus, the Greek philosopher and gynecologist, suggests as a method of emergency contraception walking energetically, riding a horse, and if that fails, to bathe in a decoction containing Wormwood to terminate the pregnancy.

WORMWOOD'S HEALING PROPERTIES

Native to Israel, the *Artemisia judaica* species is sometimes referred to as Judean Wormwood. The essential oil is extracted from the shrub by steam distillation of its leaves and flowering tops. Belonging to the Asteraceae family, Wormwood is most commonly known for its role in the production of absinthe, an alcoholic spirit that was once illegal across most of Europe.

Wormwood essential oil has a spicy, warm, bitter aroma that blends with floral, fruity oils such as Lavender, Jasmine, and Orange. It is not commonly used in modern aromatherapy.

TRADITIONAL USES

The first known use of Wormwood can be dated back to the Egyptian times when it was mentioned in a medical document in 1550 B.C. The name Wormwood is thought to be derived from its traditional use as a vermifuge – that is, expelling worms from the body.

Wormwood is described as a poison in the Bible and used as a metaphor in the Old Testament to symbolize sorrow and bitterness. As the serpent left the Garden of Eden, Wormwood is said to have sprung up along its path (Source: Hideous Absinthe: A History of the Devil in a bottle, Adams, J.). In addition, it is believed the drink Jesus was offered on the cross was a bitter blend of Wormwood and vinegar.

The ancient Greek mathematician Pythagorus recommended Wormwood as a remedy to ease labor pains. Wormwood has a long history throughout the ages of use as an aphrodisiac, digestive aid, and cure for drunkenness. The bitter taste of Wormwood was even recommended as an effective method to wean babies from breastfeeding. During the 1800s, Wormwood was used as a cheap substitute for quinine to counteract fever and dysentery among French soldiers fighting in Africa.

MEDICINAL USES

Traditionally, Wormwood was most commonly used as a remedy to treat digestive and menstrual problems. Wormwood essential oil is not generally recommended for therapeutic use in modern aromatherapy.

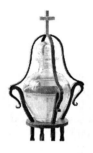

Essential Oil
DATASHEETS

Essential Oil Datasheet

Acacia Shittah (*Acacia arabica*)

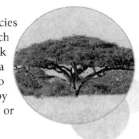

With over 1,300 varieties of Acacia, this species refers to the Shittah tree – the wood of which was used to build the Tabernacle and the Ark of the Covenant. Some believe this Acacia tree was the 'burning bush' used by God to communicate with Moses. It is also known by the name of Acacia Arabica, Acacia Nilotica or Mimosa Arabica, among others.

- **Country of Origin:** Egypt
- **Extraction Method:** Solvent Extraction
- **Plant Parts:** Flowers
- **Botanical Family:** Fabaceae
- **Chemical Families:** Menthol and limonene
- **Aroma:** Sweet, woody, balsamic, floral
- **Blends Well With:** Lavender, Ylang Ylang, Citronella, Frankincense, Orange, Cassia
- **Note:** Base

Precautions

☑ Avoid during pregnancy

Therapeutic Properties

Acacia arabica has antiseptic, antimicrobial, antiviral, demulcent and astringent properties, which make it useful for treating skin conditions and infections. It is also thought to be an aphrodisiac, due to its stimulating and energizing effects. Acacia is also an antioxidant, antidiarrheal and contains an anti-inflammatory agent.

antimicrobial	astringent	demulcent
aphrodisiac	antidiarrheal	antiseptic
anti-inflammatory	antioxidant	antiviral

Uses

- **Digestive:** Indigestion, diarrhea
- **Cardiovascular:** High cholesterol
- **Mental/Emotional:** Stress, anxiety, nervous tension, depression
- **Genito-Urinary:** Urinary infections
- **Reproductive:** Gonorrhea, leucorrhea
- **Respiratory:** Sore throats, coughs, colds, pneumonia
- **Skin:** Sores, toothache, oily skin, inflammation

Application

Acacia essential oil is generally safe to use and may be handled in the same way as other common essential oils – diffused, inhaled, added to baths or topically applied to the affected area.

Cautions

Acacia essential oil should be avoided during pregnancy. Otherwise, general essential oil safety guidelines apply.

Essential Oil Datasheet

Agarwood (*Aquilaria malaccensis*)

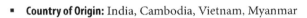

Agarwood is the resinous heartwood of large, evergreen Aquilaria trees. The fragrance develops when fungi infect the tree, producing an aromatic resin that saturates the wood. Also known as Oud or Aloeswood, this rare and expensive essential oil is referenced in ancient Indian scriptures. It is regarded as the most expensive incense in the world and highly prized in perfumery.

- **Country of Origin:** India, Cambodia, Vietnam, Myanmar
- **Extraction Method:** Steam Distillation or Hydro-Distillation
- **Plant Parts:** Agarwood chips
- **Botanical Family:** Thymelaeaceae
- **Chemical Families:** Sesquiterpenes and phenyl ethyl chromones
- **Aroma:** Sweet, balsamic, woody
- **Blends Well With:** Sandalwood, Frankincense, Rose, Neroli, Jasmine, Vetiver, Geranium
- **Note:** Base

Precautions

☑ No specific safety precautions – general essential oil guidelines apply

Therapeutic Properties

Agarwood is well known for its use as an aphrodisiac, due to its ability to stimulate the pineal gland and the limbic region of the brain, our emotional center. It is also considered to have carminative, tonic, diuretic, antimicrobial and anti-asthmatic properties.

Agarwood is known to support the nerves and circulation and has the ability to stimulate the pineal gland and the limbic region of the brain, the center of emotions. Aloes can be used for depression and meditation.

This oil can be used for bronchitis, cystitis, skin tumors, urinary tract infections, acne, pulmonary infections, menstrual problems, nervous tension, and skin conditions.

aphrodisiac	tonic	diuretic
carminative	antimicrobial	anti-asthmatic

Uses

- **Reproductive:** Can regulate menstrual disorders
- **Mental/Emotional:** Stimulates the pineal gland and limbic region of the brain, which is the center of emotions. Can ease depression and calm the mind, releasing nervous tension, stress and anxiety. Often used as an aphrodisiac.
- **Genito-Urinary:** Can be used to treat urinary tract infections, such as cystitis
- **Respiratory:** May be used to treat bronchitis
- **Nervous:** Supports the nervous system
- **Skin:** Can help to heal skin conditions, including acne, infections, and skin tumors

Application

Agarwood essential oil may be applied topically to the skin or affected area, or used in baths, compresses, diffusers, and inhalations. It can also be diffused or inhaled to treat respiratory conditions.

Cautions

Agarwood is considered to be a non-toxic oil and safe to use in aromatherapy. No specific safety precautions apply.

Essential Oil Datasheet

Anise (*Pimpinella anisum*)

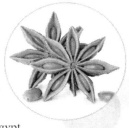

Anise is derived from an annual herb and known for its distinctive Aniseed-like aroma. It should not be confused with Star Anise, which belongs to a different family.

- **Country of Origin:** Native to Greece and Egypt
- **Extraction Method:** Steam Distillation
- **Plant Parts:** Seeds
- **Botanical Family:** Apiaceae
- **Chemical Families:** Anise is 90% anethole, which gives its distinctive aroma
- **Aroma:** Rich, spicy-sweet, licorice scent
- **Blends Well With:** Cardamom, Caraway, Cedarwood, Coriander, Dill, Fennel, Mandarin, Petitgrain, Rosewood
- **Note:** Top

Precautions

- ☑ Avoid during pregnancy
- ☑ Should not be used with estrogen-dependent cancers
- ☑ Use with caution on sensitive skin
- ☑ In large doses, Anise can have a narcotic effect and slow the circulation
- ☑ Use sparingly on children

Therapeutic Properties

Anise is useful for treating digestive disorders, due to its antispasmodic, aperient, carminative, digestive, laxative, stomachic and vermifuge properties. It is also an excellent antiseptic, decongestant and expectorant, which makes it good for respiratory problems.

Anise may be a sedative or a stimulant, depending on the dosage given. It is also an anti-epileptic, antihysteric, antirheumatic, cordial, galactagogue and insecticide.

anti-epileptic	antihysteric	antirheumatic
antiseptic	antispasmodic	aperient

carminative	cordial	decongestant
digestive	expectorant	galactagogue
insecticide	laxative	sedative
stimulant	stomachic	vermifuge

Uses

Since biblical times, Anise has been used as a domestic spice and flavoring for food and beverages. It was also traditionally used to aid digestion and freshen the breath.

Today, it is widely utilized in the pharmaceutical industry as a fragrance and/or flavoring for cough mixtures, lozenges, and dental products. In aromatherapy, it is most commonly used for digestive and respiratory ailments.

- **Digestive:** Flatulence, constipation, indigestion, stomach gas, intestinal worms, colic
- **Reproductive:** Aphrodisiac, may also help to promote the production of breast milk, menstrual cramps, may also be used to stimulate menstruation
- **Mental/Emotional:** Anxiety, stress, depression, anger
- **Muscular/Joints:** Muscular aches and pains, rheumatism, spasms, cramps
- **Respiratory:** Bronchitis, coughs, colds, flu, congestion, asthma, catarrh
- **Nervous:** Epileptic seizures, hysteria, vertigo, migraines
- **Skin:** Wounds, head lice

Application

Use in a diffuser to treat respiratory problems, or add a few drops to a handkerchief to ease migraines and digestive problems. For muscular aches and pains, dilute with a carrier oil and massage into the affected area.

Cautions

Anise should be avoided during pregnancy. It should not be used with estrogen-dependent cancers. Always use with caution on sensitive skin, and sparingly on children. In large doses, Anise can have a narcotic effect and slow the circulation.

Essential Oil Datasheet

Balsam (*Commiphora opobalsamum*)

There are several different varieties of Balsam that are used in aromatherapy. This type derives from the *Commiphora opobalsamum* bush, which produces a fragrant resin that was a traditional herbal remedy in ancient times.

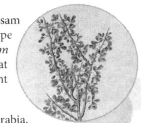

- **Country of Origin:** Egypt, Saudi Arabia, Ethiopia and Sudan
- **Extraction Method:** Dry distillation of the crude resin
- **Plant Parts:** Resin
- **Botanical Family:** Burseraceae
- **Chemical Families:** The main components of the plant are cadinol, calacorene and terpinen-4-ol
- **Aroma:** Sweet, woody, balsamic scent
- **Blends Well With:** Pine, Cedarwood, Benzoin, Lavender, Spruce, Frankincense, Lemon, Rosemary
- **Note:** Base

Precautions

☑ Generally non-toxic, although may cause skin sensitization if used in large quantities

Therapeutic Properties

Balsam is naturally antiseptic, analgesic, astringent, carminative, digestive and hypotensive. It is also an effective antioxidant and expectorant.

antiseptic	analgesic	antioxidant
astringent	carminative	digestive
expectorant	hypotensive	

Uses

- **Digestive:** Indigestion, flatulence
- **Reproductive:** Infertility
- **Muscular/Joints:** Muscular aches and pains, rheumatism, headaches, sprains
- **Respiratory:** Colds, coughs, catarrh, fever, tonsillitis, bronchitis, laryngitis
- **Immune:** Bacterial infections
- **Circulatory:** High blood pressure
- **Skin:** Bites, wounds, sores, eczema, ulcers

Application

Balsam is traditionally applied as a healing balm (or salve) for the treatment of wounds, but may also be used in massage oils, compresses, and baths. A few drops inhaled on a handkerchief can be helpful for treating respiratory conditions. Usually, herbalists prescribed a Balm of Gilead tincture (to be taken orally) to cure tonsillitis, bronchitis, and laryngitis.

Cautions

Balsam is considered to be non-toxic, although skin sensitization may occur when used in large quantities.

Essential Oil Datasheet

Bay Laurel (*Laurilus nobilis*)

Bay Laurel is a versatile oil derived from the Evergreen Laurel tree – most well known for its leaves, which are a favorite culinary ingredient in all cuisines. The essential oil from the plant is most commonly used to treat muscular aches, respiratory problems, and digestive complaints.

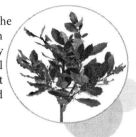

- **Country of Origin:** Mediterranean
- **Extraction Method:** Steam Distillation
- **Plant Parts:** Leaves and branches
- **Botanical Family:** Lauraceae
- **Chemical Families:** Mainly cineol (also known as eucalyptol)
- **Aroma:** Spicy, medicinal scent
- **Blends Well With:** Pine, Cypress, Juniper, Rosemary, Clary Sage, Lavender and spice oils
- **Note:** Top

Precautions

- ☑ Avoid during pregnancy
- ☑ Use with extreme care, in very low dilutions
- ☑ Potentially narcotic effects
- ☑ May cause dermal irritation or skin sensitization

Therapeutic Properties

Bay Laurel contains analgesic, antirheumatic, antiseptic, astringent, bactericidal, digestive, diuretic, emmenagogue, expectorant, fungicidal, hypotensive, sedative and stomachic properties.

analgesic	antirheumatic	antiseptic
astringent	bactericidal	digestive
diuretic	emmenagogue	expectorant
fungicidal	hypotensive	sedative
stomachic		

Uses

- **Digestive:** Indigestion, flatulence, loss of appetite
- **Menstrual:** Amenorrhea, scanty periods
- **Circulatory:** High blood pressure, fluid retention
- **Muscular/Joints:** Arthritis, rheumatism, muscular aches and pains, headaches
- **Respiratory:** Colds, flu, tonsillitis, viral infections, catarrh
- **Lymphatic:** Accumulation of toxins
- **Mental/Emotional:** Insomnia
- **Skin:** Bruises, fungal infections

Application

Apply topically to the affected area, or add 1-2 drops to a bath or warm compress. Inhale from a handkerchief to treat respiratory conditions. Bay Laurel essential oil is not recommended for internal use.

The analgesic effect of Bay Laurel makes it an excellent muscle rub when applied topically to cramps, sprains, rheumatism, and arthritis. It can also be used sparingly in compresses, diffusers, and baths.

In the past, some advocated drinking Bay Laurel tea to relieve stomach upsets or help insomnia, although it is not usually recommended for internal use.

Cautions

Bay Laurel should be avoided during pregnancy. It must be used with extreme care and in very low dilutions as it has potentially narcotic effects and may cause dermal irritation or sensitization.

Essential Oil Datasheet

Bdellium (*Commiphora africana*)

Bdellium is a species of Myrrh, commonly known as African Myrrh. Often used as an inexpensive alternative to true Myrrh, Bdellium has a long history of medicinal use. It is produced from the aromatic resin of the Commiphora Africana tree.

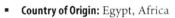

- **Country of Origin:** Egypt, Africa
- **Extraction Method:** Steam Distillation
- **Plant Parts:** Resin
- **Botanical Family:** Burseraceae
- **Chemical Families:** Mainly α-thujene, α- and β-pinene, and p-cymene
- **Aroma:** Bitter, balsamic, spicy scent that is similar to Myrrh
- **Blends Well With:** Myrrh, Benzoin, Frankincense, Lavender, Sandalwood, Clove, Patchouli
- **Note:** Base

Precautions

☑ Avoid during pregnancy

☑ May be toxic in large doses

Therapeutic Properties

Bdellium is commonly used to treat skin conditions and infections, due to its anti-inflammatory, antimicrobial, antiseptic, astringent and fungicidal properties. It can also ease digestive complaints as it has carminative, stimulant, stomachic and tonic effects on the body. As an emmenagogue, Bdellium can help with irregular or painful menstruation. It also acts as an expectorant and sedative.

anti-inflammatory	antimicrobial	antiseptic
astringent	carminative	emmenagogue
expectorant	fungicidal	sedative
stimulant	stomachic	tonic

Uses

- **Digestive:** Diarrhea, indigestion, flatulence, loss of appetite
- **Menstrual:** Amenorrhea, dysmenorrhea
- **Mental/Emotional:** Emotionally balancing
- **Muscular/Joints:** Arthritis
- **Respiratory:** Coughs, colds, catarrh, sore throat, asthma
- **Skin:** Aging skin, sun-damaged skin, acne, wounds, dry skin, fungal infections, and sores

Application

Bdellium essential oil may be diffused, inhaled, added to baths or applied topically to the affected area.

Cautions

Bdellium should not be used during pregnancy, and may be toxic in large doses.

Essential Oil Datasheet

Calamus (*Acorus calamus*)

The scented leaves and rhizomes of the Calamus plant are used to produce the aromatic essential oil, which has a long history of use as a perfume and medicinal remedy. The perennial plant prefers lake margins, swampy ditches, or protected marshes.

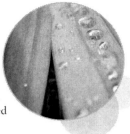

- **Country of Origin:** India
- **Extraction Method:** Steam Distillation
- **Plant Parts:** Rhizomes
- **Botanical Family:** Araceae
- **Chemical Families:** Beta-asarone, calamene, calamol, calamenene, eugenol and shyobunones
- **Aroma:** Medium, refreshing scent, similar to Cinnamon
- **Blends Well With:** Lavender, Tea Tree, Rosemary, Clary Sage, Geranium, Marjoram
- **Note:** Base

Precautions

- ☑ Avoid during pregnancy
- ☑ Large doses can cause mild hallucinations and narcotic effects
- ☑ Contains asarone, which is potentially toxic (and may be carcinogenic)
- ☑ Avoid oral ingestion, which can cause prolonged severe convulsions and tumors

Therapeutic Properties

Calamus is a stimulating nervine, antispasmodic and tonic oil. Being antirheumatic and anti-arthritic, it is a useful oil for treating aches and pains. As a stimulant, it boosts the circulation, which can bring relief from painful inflammation. It is also effective for fighting bacteria, parasites, and infectious conditions, with antiseptic, bactericidal, insecticide and vermifuge properties. As a hypotensive, it can lower the blood pressure. Although Calamus is classed as a stimulant, in small doses it may be used as a sedative to calm the mind and induce sleep. As a stimulant for the brain and nervous system, it is used to promote cerebral circulation, to stimulate self-expression, and to help manage a broad range of symptoms in the head, including neuralgia, epilepsy, memory loss, and shock. Acorus Calamus shows a neuroprotective effect against stroke and chemically induced neurodegeneration in the rat. Specifically, it has a protective effect against acrylamide-induced neurotoxicity.

nervine	antispasmodic	tonic
stimulant	antirheumatic	anti-arthritic
sedative	antiseptic	bactericidal
carminative	diaphoretic	expectorant
hypotensive	insecticide	vermifuge

Uses

- **Mental/Emotional:** Stimulates the brain helps with memory loss, shock, and self-expression. It also helps to promote positive thoughts. Its memory-boosting properties can help to repair damaged brain tissues and neurons. In small doses, it can help to relax the body and induce sleep.

- **Circulation:** May be used to stimulate the circulation, particularly in the brain.

- **Muscular/Joints:** Provides relief from pain and swelling associated with rheumatism, arthritis, gout and muscular spasms.

- **Immune:** Acts as an antibiotic against internal and external infections.

- **Nervous:** Refreshes and stimulates the nervous system and helps with neuralgia, epilepsy, nervous spasms and neurotic disorders. It helps to contract blood vessels to reduce pressure on the cranial nerve, which relieves pain from neuralgia and headaches. Studies on rats have proven it to have a neuroprotective effect against strokes and neurodegeneration. It also has a protective effect against acrylamide-induced neurotoxicity.

Application

Calamus can be inhaled from the bottle, applied to the abdomen, or on location for soothing and calming effects. Uses for Calamus oil include inhalations, diffusers, and baths or applied directly to the affected area.

Caution

Caution is advised on the use of this essential oil since large doses can cause mild hallucinations. The essential oil in the roots of this plant contains the compound asarone. This has tranquilizing and antibiotic activity but is also potentially toxic. Use well diluted. It has narcotic effects and can cause convulsions and hallucinations if taken in higher doses. Studies have shown that its oral ingestion can cause prolonged severe convulsions and tumors. So, oral ingestion should be avoided unless under the guidance of an expert practitioner. Avoid during pregnancy.

Essential Oil Datasheet

Cassia (*Cinnamomum cassia*)

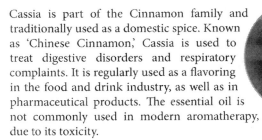

Cassia is part of the Cinnamon family and traditionally used as a domestic spice. Known as 'Chinese Cinnamon,' Cassia is used to treat digestive disorders and respiratory complaints. It is regularly used as a flavoring in the food and drink industry, as well as in pharmaceutical products. The essential oil is not commonly used in modern aromatherapy, due to its toxicity.

- **Country of Origin:** China
- **Extraction Method:** Steam Distillation
- **Plant Parts:** Leaves, bark, twigs and stalks
- **Botanical Family:** Lauraceae
- **Chemical Families:** Mainly cinnamic aldehyde (75-90%)
- **Aroma:** Pungent, sweet, woody, spicy
- **Blends Well With:** Benzoin, Clove Bud, Coriander, Cardamom, Frankincense, Ginger, Grapefruit, Lavender, Rosemary, Thyme
- **Note:** Top

Precautions

☑ Dermal toxin and irritant – should only be used in very low dilutions and with extreme care

☑ May irritate mucous membranes if directly inhaled

Therapeutic Properties

Cassia is an excellent oil for treating infections, as it provides antibacterial, antiviral, antifungal, astringent and antimicrobial properties. For digestive-related problems, it is anti-inflammatory, anti-emetic, carminative and antidiarrheal. Cassia is also considered to be an emmenagogue, a stimulant, an anticoagulant and a febrifuge.

antibacterial	antiviral	antifungal
anti-inflammatory	anticoagulant	anti-emetic
antimicrobial	astringent	carminative

antidiarrheal	antidepressant	antirheumatic
emmenagogue	febrifuge	stimulant

Uses

- **Digestive:** Useful for treating diarrhea, nausea, gas, vomiting and intestinal infections
- **Circulatory:** Stimulates the circulation
- **Menstrual:** Eases painful periods and regulates the menstrual cycle
- **Immune:** Supports the immune system, boosts the body's natural defenses and is effective at fighting bacteria, viruses, and fungal infections.
- **Muscular/Joints:** Brings warmth and relief to stiff joints, rheumatism and arthritis
- **Mental/Emotional:** Uplifts the spirits, helps with depression
- **Respiratory:** Fights coughs, colds, flu and viral infections. Helps to lower body temperature during a fever.
- **Skin:** Soothes dry, sensitive skin. Can be used to treat fungal skin and nail infections.

Application

Cassia oil may be used in a diffuser, or applied topically to the skin if well diluted with a carrier oil. Dilute 1 part essential oil with 4 parts carrier oil and apply one to two drops on location; diffuse, or burn in incense. Boost your immunity against infections by inhaling the essential oil or rubbing it over the soles of your feet.

Cautions

Cassia oil is classed as a dermal toxin and irritant, so it should always be used with extreme care. Do not inhale directly, as it can irritate mucous membranes. Use Cassia oil in very low dilutions and avoid using on very sensitive skin. This oil can be warming to the skin so be sure to dilute with a carrier oil.

Essential Oil Datasheet

Cedarwood (*Cedrus atlantica*)

Cedarwood has been traditionally for bronchitis, urinary tract infections, as a preservative and as incense. Other varieties of Cedarwood include Virginian Cedarwood (*Juniperus virginiana*), Texas Cedarwood (*Juniperus mexicana*), and Himalayan Cedarwood (*Cedrus deodara*).

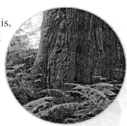

- **Country of Origin:** Native to the Atlas Mountains of Algeria, produced mainly in Morocco.
- **Extraction Method:** Steam Distillation, with small quantities produced by absolutes
- **Plant Parts:** Wood stumps and sawdust of trees
- **Botanical Family:** Pinaceae, Cupressaceae
- **Chemical Families:** Sesquiterpenes, sesquiterpenols
- **Aroma:** balsamic, sweet, woody
- **Note:** Base

Precautions

- ☑ Check for allergies with Cedarwood
- ☑ *Cedrus atlantica* is not for children under 5; others are fine
- ☑ Avoid with the history of estrogen-dependent cancer

Therapeutic Properties

aphrodisiac	antibacterial	antidepressant
antifungal	astringent	antiseptic
antiviral	circulatory stimulant	diuretic
expectorant	insecticide	mucolytic
sedative	tonic	vulnerary

Uses

☑ **Circulation:** arthritis, rheumatism, and fluid retention.

☑ **Mental/Emotional:** brings harmony to the nervous system, calming, soothing, assists with concentration and mental clarity. Counters nervous tension, depression, anxiety, exhaustion, and stress-related conditions.

☑ **Respiratory:** treats excess phlegm, asthma, bronchitis, colds, brings relief for coughs, and respiratory complaints.

☑ **Urinary:** treats urinary, kidney, bladder complaints, infections, and cystitis.

☑ **Skin/Hair:** effective for acne, dermatitis, eczema, fungal infections, cuts, insect repellant, wounds, hair care, dandruff, greasy hair, and alopecia areata (hair loss).

Application

Diffuse or use topically on location.

Cautions

Cedarwood is considered non-toxic and non-irritant. Avoid during pregnancy.

Essential Oil Datasheet

Cinnamon Bark (*Cinnamomum zeylanicum*)

Two different types of essential oil are extracted from the Cinnamon plant. Cinnamon Leaf, which is more commonly used for therapeutic purposes in aromatherapy and Cinnamon Bark oil, which is not generally recommended for use on the skin. Both are used for fragrance and flavoring in food, drinks, toiletries and pharmaceutical products.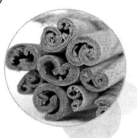

- **Country of Origin:** China, Southeast Asia, India
- **Extraction Method:** Steam Distillation
- **Plant Parts:** Bark
- **Botanical Family:** Lauraceae
- **Chemical Families:** Mainly cinnamaldehyde (40-50%), eugenol and others
- **Aroma:** Warm, pleasant, spicy scent
- **Blends Well With:** Frankincense, Orange, Lemon, Rosemary, Lavender, Benzoin
- **Note:** Base-Middle

Precautions

☑ Dermal toxin and irritant – use with extreme care

☑ May irritate mucous membranes if directly inhaled

Therapeutic Properties

antimicrobial	anti-infectious	antibacterial
antiseptic	anti-inflammatory	antiviral
antifungal	anticoagulant	antidepressant
antidiarrheal	antispasmodic	aphrodisiac
astringent	carminative	digestive
emmenagogue	stimulant	stomachic

Uses

- **Digestive:** Calms spasms of the digestive tract, indigestion, diarrhea, colitis, vomiting and nausea
- **Circulatory:** Helps to reduce blood pressure, improves the circulation
- **Menstrual:** Regulates scanty periods
- **Mental/Emotional:** Cinnamon has the ability to lift the spirits and is an effective treatment for depression, nervous exhaustion, and stress-related conditions
- **Immune:** Boosts the immune system and combats viral, bacterial and fungal infections
- **Respiratory:** Has the ability to fight viral respiratory conditions, including influenza
- **Skin:** Heals fungal skin and nail infections, stings, scabies and lice
- **Endocrine:** Can be used to treat diabetes and high blood sugar

Application

Cinnamon Bark oil may be diffused or applied topically to the skin – however, you must ensure it is well diluted in a carrier oil due to its high phenol content (1 drop essential oil to 40-50 drops carrier oil). Alternatively, use Cinnamon Leaf oil, which offers the same medicinal properties while relatively non-toxic. Cinnamon may be used in food or beverage as a dietary supplement (0-size capsule).

Cautions

This oil may be a potent skin irritant (skin may turn red or burn). Because of its high phenol content, it is best diluted (1 drop to 40 or 50 drops of a carrier oil, such as extra-virgin Olive oil) before applying to the skin. If the mixture is too hot, apply additional diluting oil. Use extreme care as it may irritate the nasal membranes if inhaled directly from diffuser or bottle. Avoid during pregnancy.

Essential Oil Datasheet

Coriander (*Coriandrum sativum*)

Widely used as a culinary herb, Coriander is also an excellent essential oil in aromatherapy. Its sweet, spicy scent combines well with other oils, making it an excellent addition to blends for muscular or digestive problems, among others.

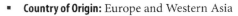

- **Country of Origin:** Europe and Western Asia
- **Extraction Method:** Steam Distillation
- **Plant Parts:** Seeds
- **Botanical Family:** Apiaceae
- **Chemical Families:** Mainly linalool
- **Aroma:** Sweet, spicy, musky scent
- **Blends Well With:** Clary Sage, Bergamot, Jasmine, Neroli, Sandalwood, Cypress, Pine and spice oils
- **Note:** Middle

Precautions

☑ Generally non-toxic and non-irritant
☑ Use with moderation – can be stupefying in large doses

Therapeutic Properties

Coriander is useful for aromatherapy blends aimed at the digestive system, due to its antispasmodic, aperitif, digestive, carminative and stomachic properties. It is also analgesic and antirheumatic, which helps with muscular pain. Other properties include aphrodisiac, antioxidant, bactericidal, depurative and fungicidal.

analgesic	aperitif	aphrodisiac
antioxidant	antirheumatic	antispasmodic
bactericidal	depurative	digestive
carminative	cytotoxic	fungicidal
lipolytic	stimulant	stomachic

Uses

- **Digestive:** Loss of appetite, colic, diarrhea, indigestion, flatulence, nausea, spasms, piles
- **Circulatory:** Fluid retention, poor circulation
- **Lymphatic:** Accumulation of toxins
- **Muscular/Joints:** Arthritis, gout, muscular aches and pains, rheumatism, cramps
- **Respiratory:** Colds, flu, infections, measles
- **Nervous:** Nervous exhaustion, debility, migraines, neuralgia
- **Mental/Emotional:** Stress, depression

Application

Coriander oil can be diffused, inhaled, added to baths or applied topically to the affected area.

Cautions

Although Coriander is generally non-toxic and non-irritating, it should be used with moderation. In large doses, Coriander can have a stupefying effect – leading to nausea, fatigue, and confusion.

Essential Oil Datasheet

Cumin (*Cuminum cyminum*)

Cumin is particularly beneficial for the digestive and nervous systems. Its spicy, warming aroma soothes muscular problems while stimulating the digestive system.

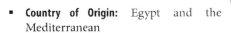

- **Country of Origin:** Egypt and the Mediterranean
- **Extraction Method:** Steam Distillation
- **Plant Parts:** Seeds
- **Botanical Family:** Apiaceae
- **Chemical Families:** Mainly aldehydes and monoterpene hydrocarbons
- **Aroma:** Warm, sensual, spicy
- **Blends Well With:** Lavender, Rosemary, Rosewood, Cardamom and other spice oils
- **Note:** Middle-Base

Precautions

☑ Avoid during pregnancy

☑ Phototoxic – avoid exposure to sunlight or UV light

Therapeutic Properties

Cumin is well known for its ability to help with gastrointestinal disorders, due to its digestive, depurative, carminative, antispasmodic, stimulant and tonic properties. It is also antiseptic and bactericidal, which helps to fight bacterial infections. Other properties include antioxidant, aphrodisiac, diuretic, nervine and emmenagogue.

antioxidant	antiseptic	antispasmodic
antitoxic	aphrodisiac	bactericidal
carminative	depurative	digestive
diuretic	emmenagogue	larvicidal
nervine	stimulant	tonic

Uses

- **Digestive:** Colic, indigestion, flatulence, spasms, constipation
- **Lymphatic:** Accumulation of toxins
- **Muscular/Joints:** Headaches, arthritis, aches, and pains
- **Nervous:** Debility, migraines, nervous exhaustion
- **Circulatory:** Poor circulation, fluid retention

Application

Cumin essential oil may be diffused, inhaled or used in baths, massage oils or applied topically to the affected area. It is advisable to use Cumin in small quantities, as its scent can be overpowering.

Cautions

As an emmenagogue, Cumin should be avoided during pregnancy. Although generally non-irritating, it is a phototoxic oil – so one should avoid exposure to the sun or UV light for 24-48 hours after application.

Essential Oil Datasheet

Cypress (*Cupressus sempervirens*)

The use of Cypress dates back thousands of years from ancient cultures such as the Egyptians, Hebrews, Greeks, and Romans. The name "sempervirens" means everlasting, as it was dedicated to the gods of the underworld – hence, why Cypress trees were grown in cemeteries. It is considered a significant oil to be used in times of transition, such as with career changes, relocating, ending a relationship, or death. This oil is quite grounding and breathtaking.

- **Country of Origin:** Native to eastern Mediterranean, distillation and cultivation is done in France, Spain, and Morocco.
- **Extraction Method:** Steam Distillation
- **Plant Parts:** Leaves, Twigs, and Cones
- **Botanical Family:** Cupressaceae
- **Chemical Families:** Monoterpenes
- **Aroma:** outdoorsy, balsamic, piney, woodsy
- **Blends Well With:** Bergamot, Clary Sage, Lavender, Juniper, Pine, Marjoram, Sandalwood, Rosemary, Frankincense and all the citrus oils.
- **Note:** Middle-Base

Precautions

- ☑ Avoid use with a history of estrogen-dependent cancer
- ☑ Avoid during pregnancy
- ☑ Non-toxic, non-irritating, and non-sensitizing.

Therapeutic Properties

The uses of Cypress are numerous. Recent research shows it is beneficial for cellulite, edema, poor circulation, and muscular cramps.

antibacterial	antifungal	antirheumatic
antiviral	antiseptic	antispasmodic
astringent	deodorant	diuretic

hepatic	sudorific	tonic
vasoconstrictive		

Uses

Cypress helps with inflammation, prevents and/or relieves chronic rheumatic pain and swelling, contracts and tightens tissue, reduces nasal mucus production and swelling and aids in the reduction of fluids, and as a tonic, strengthens and restores vitality. Cypress influences, strengthens and helps ease the feeling of loss. It creates a feeling of security and grounding, helping to heal emotional trauma.

- **Circulation:** aids in cellulite, muscular cramps, edema, poor circulation, and rheumatism, muscle spasms, and fluid retention.
- **Menstruation:** menopausal complaints, excessive menstruation, stimulates estrogen secretions, relieves painful periods, and dysmenorrheal.
- **Mental/Emotional:** good for the nervous system, tension, and stress-related symptoms, depression, calming and soothing, counters anxiety, and insomnia. Soothes excessive talking, overthinking and feeling of being overwhelmed. Eases major life transitions and assists with the grieving process.
- **Muscular/Joints:** treats rheumatic pain, back pain, muscular aches and pains, and arthritis.
- **Respiration:** treats asthma, bronchitis, chills, colic, coughs, laryngitis, and issues with the mucous membrane.
- **Skin:** helps with hemorrhoids, oily skin, excessive perspiration, insect repellent, bleeding of the gums, varicose veins, and wounds that won't heal.

Application

Use topically on location. Apply where you would wear a deodorant.

Cautions

This oil is considered non-toxic, non-irritating, and can be used by most. If oxidized, it may cause skin irritation or sensitization. Some sources recommend avoiding Cypress essential oil during pregnancy, but there is no research to support this statement.

Essential Oil Datasheet

Dill (*Anethum graveolens*)

The fresh scent of Dill is stimulating, revitalizing and balancing. Its soothing nature makes it an effective digestive aid, as well as a remedy to calm the mind.

- **Country of Origin:** Mediterranean and the Black Sea
- **Extraction Method:** Steam Distillation
- **Plant Parts:** Seeds
- **Botanical Family:** Apiaceae
- **Chemical Families:** Mainly carvone (30-60%) plus limonene, eugenol, pinene and others. There are several different chemotypes of Dill so chemical constituents will vary.
- **Aroma:** Fresh, sweet, grassy fragrance
- **Blends Well With:** Elemi, Mint, Caraway, Nutmeg, Bergamot, citrus and spice oils
- **Note:** Middle

Precautions

- ☑ Dill is generally non-toxic and non-irritant
- ☑ As an emmenagogue, it is not advisable to use Dill during pregnancy

Therapeutic Properties

Dill is mainly beneficial for digestive disorders, due to its antispasmodic, carminative, digestive and stomachic properties. Other therapeutic properties include bactericidal, emmenagogue, galactagogue, hypotensive and stimulant.

antispasmodic	bactericidal	carminative
digestive	emmenagogue	galactagogue
hypotensive	stimulant	stomachic

Uses

- **Digestive:** Colic, indigestion, flatulence, constipation, bloating, cramps, bad breath
- **Menstrual:** Amenorrhea, dysmenorrhea
- **Reproductive:** Promotes the production of breast milk
- **Mental/Emotional:** Stress, nervous tension, insomnia
- **Circulatory:** High blood pressure
- **Immune:** Bacterial infections
- **Endocrine:** Can stabilize blood sugar
- **Nervous:** Hiccups
- **Skin:** Wounds

Application

For digestive problems or menstrual cramps, it is most effective when massaged into the abdomen area. The oil can also be diffused, inhaled or used in baths.

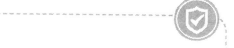

Cautions

Dill is an emmenagogue, so it is best avoided during pregnancy. Otherwise, it is generally non-toxic and non-irritating.

Essential Oil Datasheet

Fennel, Sweet (*Foeniculum vulgare dulce*)

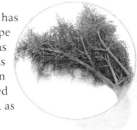

Sweet Fennel is an erect perennial herb has yellow flowers, is native to Southern Europe and can reach up to 4.5 feet. The plant has yellow flowers. Bitter Fennel was known as fenkle in the Middle Ages, from the Latin *foenum* meaning "hay." The ancients believed it gave one longevity, courage and strength, as well as warded off evil spirits.

- **Country of Origin:** Southern Europe
- **Extraction Method:** Steam Distillation
- **Plant Parts:** Seeds
- **Botanical Family:** Umbelliferae
- **Chemical Families:** Monoterpenes, ketones, esters
- **Aroma:** Exotic and sensual, herbaceous, sweet, warm and radiant
- **Note:** Middle

Precautions

- ☑ Phototoxic
- ☑ May cause skin irritation in some individuals
- ☑ Avoid contact with eyes

Therapeutic Properties

Fennel essential oil has been found to aid with digestion and helps to relieve flatulence, indigestion, and digestive discomfort. Sweet Fennel contains the chemical trans-anethole (ether) and should not be used by pregnant or breastfeeding women.

antiemetic	antispasmodic	carminative
diuretic	emmenagogue	expectorant
tonic	antiseptic	analgesic

Uses

- **Bones/Joints:** Gout
- **Circulatory:** Supports the heart
- **Digestive:** Promotes digestion, reduces indigestion, expels worms, sluggish digestion, nausea, intestinal parasites, intestinal spasms, constipation
- **Lymphatic:** Breaks up fluids and toxins; cleanses tissue
- **Mental/Emotional:** Helps with feelings of being stuck and withdrawn. Reduces tension and inhibitions with communication. Help dissolve creative blocks. Energetic protection.
- **Reproductive:** Stimulates estrogen production, facilitates birthing, increases lactation, premenstrual problems (PMS).
- **Respiratory:** Supports the respiratory system, fluid retention
- **Skin:** Antiseptic

Application

Use in compresses or massage oils to reduce swelling, in particular using with lymphatic drainage massage. Use Fennel tea bags to reduce puffy eyes. Abdominal massage with Fennel oil will aid digestion and also reduce a little one's gripes from colic.

Cautions

Fennel oil is strong. It is probably the most powerful of all the diuretics, and for this reason, it should be avoided during pregnancy.

This essential oil has phototoxic properties, and exposure to the sun should be avoided after application to the skin. Dilute well before use; for external use only. May cause skin irritation in some individuals; a skin test is recommended before use. Contact with eyes should be avoided. It should be used briefly and only at a 1% dilution.

Essential Oil Datasheet

Fir (*Abies alba*)

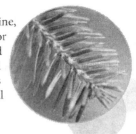

With a fresh, woody fragrance similar to Pine, Fir oil is often associated with winter or Christmas time. Fir or Fir Needle oil could refer to a variety of individual oils produced from coniferous trees. Therefore it is important to determine the specific botanical name for any given oil.

- **Country of Origin:** Northern Europe
- **Extraction Method:** Steam Distillation
- **Plant Parts:** Needles, twigs or Fir cones
- **Botanical Family:** Pinaceae
- **Chemical Families:** Santene, pinene, limonene, bornyl acetate and others
- **Aroma:** Fresh, sweet, woody, balsamic scent
- **Blends Well With:** Lavender, Rosemary, Cedarwood, Pine, Lemon and Marjoram
- **Note:** Middle

Precautions

- ☑ Generally non-toxic
- ☑ Possible irritant to sensitive skin

Therapeutic Properties

Fir essential oil is an analgesic, stimulant, and tonic, making it a good oil for treating aches and pains, poor circulation and general exhaustion. Its expectorant properties can help with respiratory problems. Fir also offers antiseptic, rubefacient and deodorant properties.

analgesic	antiseptic	deodorant
expectorant	rubefacient	stimulant
tonic		

Uses

- **Circulatory:** Poor circulation
- **Muscular/Joints:** Muscular aches and pains, rheumatism, arthritis
- **Respiratory:** Coughs, colds, flu, tonsillitis, sinusitis
- **Nervous:** Fatigue, nervous exhaustion
- **Skin:** Wounds, cuts, burns

Application

Fir oil may be diffused or inhaled to treat respiratory conditions, or applied topically to an affected area. It is not recommended for use in baths, due to its potential to irritate sensitive areas.

Cautions

Fir essential oil is generally non-toxic, although it can irritate sensitive skin.

Essential Oil Datasheet

Frankincense (*Boswellia carterii*)

Frankincense is highly prized in the aromatherapy industry. It is frequently used in skin care products as it is considered a valuable ingredient having remarkable anti-aging, rejuvenating and healing properties.

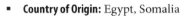

- **Country of Origin:** Egypt, Somalia
- **Extraction Method:** Steam Distillation
- **Plant Parts:** Resins/gum
- **Botanical Family:** Burseraceae
- **Chemical Families:** Monoterpenes, sesquiterpenes, sesquiterpenols, monoterpenols
- **Aroma:** Rich, woodsy, balsamic, earthy, resinous, warm
- **Note:** Base
- **Blends Well With:** Cedarwood and Cinnamon

Precautions

- ☑ Can be irritating to the skin if oxidized
- ☑ Avoid use during pregnancy

Therapeutic Properties

Frankincense is a favorite for quieting the mind and encouraging emotional healing on all levels. Some of its properties include being antimicrobial, immuno-stimulant, antidepressant, anti-inflammatory, arthritis, antiseptic, astringent, carminative, digestive, diuretic, sedative, tonic and expectorant.

analgesic	anti-inflammatory	carminative
cicatrisant	diuretic	expectorant
immuno-stimulant	skin healing	tonic

Uses

- **Mental/Emotional:** good for anxiety, depression, and nervous tension; very calming.
- **Muscular:** provides pain relief, helps with tension in neck muscles and spasms.
- **Respiratory:** helps to calm the lungs and quiet coughs, asthma, and other respiratory conditions. Good for infections.
- **Skin/Hair:** used for dry and aging skin. Good for reducing scar tissue.

Application

Diffuse or apply topically.

Caution

Non-toxic, non-irritant and can be used by most.

Essential Oil Datasheet

Galbanum (*Ferula galbaniflua*)

Galbanum is a top note essential oil that is great to help with healing wounds and is really effective towards sores and ulcers.

- **Country of Origin:** France
- **Extraction Method:** Steam Distillation
- **Plant Parts:** Resin
- **Botanical Family:** Rutaceae
- **Aroma:** Sweet
- **Note:** Top

Precautions

- ☑ Avoid during pregnancy
- ☑ Not for children under 5
- ☑ Possible skin irritant

Therapeutic Properties

anti-arthritic	antibacterial	antidepressant
antirheumatic	emollient	antiseptic
antispasmodic	antiviral	vulnerary
cicatrisant	circulatory	antioxidant
decongestant	insecticide	immune support
detoxifier	antiparasitic	disinfectant

Uses

The oil can be used in a variety of ways and helps when speeding up the healing of wounds, acne, boils and sores. Galbanum is also used to help recover from shock, trauma, and depression.

- **Respiratory:** Blood circulation
- **Menstrual:** Helps cure arthritis and rheumatism.
- **Muscular/Joints:** Muscular boils, acne, and abscesses.
- **Skin:** Rejuvenates aging skin and keeps skin healthy and shining.

Application

Diffuse or apply topically. Dilute with a carrier oil according to its use.

Cautions

No safety hazards are found; however, it should not be used in heavy dosages.

Essential Oil Datasheet

Garlic (*Allium sativum*)

Garlic is a member of the Allium family, along with onions, leeks, and chives. The perennial herb is one of the most commonly used plants in the world, known mainly for its use as a flavoring ingredient in all types of cuisines. Although not normally used in modern aromatherapy, its clear-colored essential oil can be used to treat a number of digestives, circulatory and infectious conditions.

- **Country of Origin:** Central Asia
- **Extraction Method:** Steam Distillation
- **Plant Parts:** Bulb
- **Botanical Family:** Amaryllidaceae
- **Chemical Families:** Allicin, allylpropyl disulphide, diallyl disulphide and others
- **Aroma:** Strong, distinctive, pungent garlic-like odor
- **Blends Well With:** Due to its strong scent, Garlic oil is best used on its own
- **Note:** Top

Precautions

☑ May irritate the stomach
☑ Possible skin sensitizer

Therapeutic Properties

The essential oil is steam distilled from the crushed garlic bulbs. It is a powerful insecticide, antibacterial and antifungal. It can be used on warts and corns as well as athlete's foot. Fresh Garlic (but not old or dried) has been found to be effective in the fight against E. coli.

amoebicidal	antibiotic	antimicrobial
antiseptic	antitoxic	antiviral
bactericidal	carminative	cholagogue
depurative	diaphoretic	diuretic

expectorant	febrifuge	fungicidal
hypoglycemic	hypotensive	insecticidal
larvicidal	stomachic	tonic

Uses

- **Digestive:** When taken internally, helps to settle gastro-intestinal infections and expels parasites
- **Genito-Urinary:** May be used to treat urinary tract infections, including cystitis
- **Circulatory:** Boosts the circulation, strengthens the heart, lowers blood pressure and reduces cholesterol levels
- **Immune:** Beneficial for supporting the immune system and fighting infectious conditions
- **Respiratory:** Can be used to treat bronchitis, coughs, colds, catarrh and sinusitis
- **Skin:** Helps to heal acne, scabies, scars, parasites and infectious skin conditions

Application

Garlic essential oil is not commonly used externally in aromatherapy, due to its overpowering odor. It is sometimes taken internally in the form of capsules. It is also commonly used in cookery. Never use more than one drop in any application. It is an extremely aromatic strong oil but delivers emotionally aggressive healing.

Cautions

Do not use during pregnancy.

Essential Oil Datasheet

Henna (*Lawsonia inermis*)

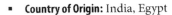

Henna leaf absolute, famous for Henna dye, is used mostly for perfumes and biblical blends. Henna leaf absolute is a very dark green paste with a deep herbaceous fragrance.

- **Country of Origin:** India, Egypt
- **Extraction Method:** Alcohol Extracted
- **Plant Parts:** Flowers, leaves, and twigs
- **Botanical Family:** Lythracoae
- **Chemical Families:** Lawsone, dehydroxyacetone
- **Aroma:** Herbaceous, tea-like bouquet, sweet licorice note
- **Note:** Middle-Base
- **Medical Properties:** Antibacterial, antitumor, emmenagogue, rejuvenating, relaxant, stimulant (hair growth). Used to induce menstruation or uterine contractions, screen the sun, clear the mind. Used for meditation and dye for the skin.
- **Blends Well With:** Neroli, Tonka Bean Absolute, Lavender, Blue Chamomile, Rose Absolute, Ylang Ylang and various spice oils.

Precautions

- ☑ Do not use with infants or children
- ☑ Avoid use during pregnancy
- ☑ Therapeutic Properties
- ☑ Cyprinum is the name of the oil extracted from Henna flowers.

antibacterial	anti-tumoral	emmenagogue
relaxant	stimulant for hair	uterine contraction
sunscreen	meditative	sharpens the mind

Uses

- **Mental/Emotional:** good for anxiety, depression, very calming and clears the mind; used for meditation.
- **Reproductive:** stimulates menstrual function or uterine contractions.
- **Skin/Hair:** used externally to treat skin diseases; serves as a dye for skin and nails. Can be used in blends to prevent infection; used for sunscreen.

Application

Can be used in the bath, for ceremonial rituals, and for massage.

Cautions

Avoid during pregnancy and with infants and children. Leaves a tint on the skin. No formal testing has been conducted.

Essential Oil Datasheet

Hyssop (*Hyssopus officinalis*)

Hyssop has a history of use as a medicinal herb since ancient times and was used to purify sacred spaces. Its name is derived from the Hebrew term '*azob*,' which means holy herb. The essential oil is mainly used to treat respiratory conditions, menstrual problems and skin disorders.

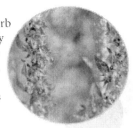

- **Country of Origin:** France, Hungary
- **Extraction Method:** Steam Distillation
- **Plant Parts:** Leaves and flowering tops
- **Botanical Family:** Lamiaceae
- **Chemical Families:** Pinocamphone, a-pinene, b-pinene, camphene, myrcene, limonene, thujone, geraniol, estragole, borneol and others
- **Aroma:** Sweet, camphor-like scent with a spicy, herbal undertone
- **Blends Well With:** Lavender, Rosemary, Bay Leaf, Clary Sage, Geranium and citrus oils
- **Note:** Middle

Precautions

☑ Avoid in epilepsy and pregnancy
☑ Moderately toxic – should only be used in moderation

Therapeutic Properties

Valerie Cooksley, R.N., wrote in her book *Aromatherapy*, the uses of Hyssop include anti-inflammatory, antioxidant, antiparasitic, antiseptic, and antiviral.

antiseptic	disinfectant	anti-infectious
anticatarrhal	decongestant	cleansing
purifying	hypertensive	diaphoretic
anti-inflammatory	antioxidant	antiparasitic

antiviral	astringent	antispasmodic
bactericidal	carminative	digestive
diuretic	emmenagogue	expectorant
febrifuge	nervine	sedative
stimulant	antirheumatic	cicatrisant
hypertensive	tonic	sudorfic
vermifuge	vulnerary	

Uses

- **Digestive:** Eases indigestion and can help to expel parasites (worms) from the digestive system
- **Circulatory:** Regulates blood pressure
- **Endocrine:** Helps to reduce fat in tissue
- **Menstrual:** Regulates absent or scanty periods
- **Mental/Emotional:** Can help anxiety, guilt, grief, insomnia, fatigue and nervous tension
- **Muscular/Joints:** Soothes the pain of arthritis and rheumatism
- **Respiratory:** May be used as a treatment for asthma, bronchitis, catarrh, coughs, colds, viral infections and sore throats
- **Nervous:** Strengthens and tones the nervous system
- **Skin:** Helps to heal wounds, bruises, cuts, scars, eczema, dermatitis and inflammation

Application

Hyssop may be diffused or applied topically to the affected area. The oil should be diluted well with a carrier oil and used in moderation.

Cautions

Avoid using if you suffer from epilepsy or are pregnant.

Essential Oil Datasheet

Juniper (*Juniperus osteosperma*)

Several varieties of Juniper essential oil are used in aromatherapy. *Juniperus osteosperma*, also known as Utah Juniper, is one variety that is native to the southwestern area of the USA.

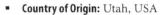

- **Country of Origin:** Utah, USA
- **Extraction Method:** Steam Distillation
- **Plant Parts:** Stems, leaves, and flowers
- **Botanical Family:** Cupressaceae
- **Chemical Families:** Alpha-Pinene (20-40%) plus camphene, bornyl acetate and others
- **Aroma:** Clear, woody, refreshing scent
- **Blends Well With:** Vetiver, Sandalwood, Cedarwood, Cypress, Pine, Fir and Lavender
- **Note:** Top-Middle

Precautions

☑ Avoid with pregnancy or kidney disease
☑ Not suitable for use on children
☑ Possible skin irritant – avoid on face and sensitive areas

Therapeutic Properties

Juniper has antibacterial, antifungal, antiviral and antimicrobial properties, making it a good oil for treating all types of infections. As an analgesic, anti-inflammatory, antirheumatic and antispasmodic oil, it is also helpful for muscular pain, cramps and inflammation. Other properties include antioxidant, antitussive, hypotensive, astringent, detoxifier, tonic and diuretic.

antibacterial	antifungal	antioxidant
anti-inflammatory	antitussive	antispasmodic
antiviral	hypotensive	antimicrobial
astringent	antirheumatic	analgesic
detoxifier	tonic	diuretic

Uses

- **Digestive:** Indigestion, gas, cramps
- **Circulatory:** Poor circulation
- **Urinary:** Supports urinary system
- **Mental/Emotional:** Stress, depression, mental fatigue, anxiety
- **Muscular/Joints:** Rheumatism
- **Respiratory:** Colds, flu, infections
- **Lymphatic:** Accumulation of toxins
- **Skin:** Aging skin, wrinkles, wounds, acne, eczema

Application

Juniper oil may be diffused, inhaled or applied topically to the affected area. It should only be used in low dilutions. Traditionally, Juniper was diffused to purify the air and treat respiratory conditions. For muscular problems, Juniper can be massaged into the affected area to relieve spasms, pain, and stiffness. Always use in moderation.

Cautions

As a potential skin irritant, Juniper should not be used on sensitive areas. It should also be avoided by children, pregnant women and those with kidney disease.

Essential Oil Datasheet

Marjoram, Sweet (*Origanum marjorana*)

Sweet Marjoram, not to be confused with "Spanish Marjoram," is a part of the Origanum family. This camphoraceous essential oil is high in the constituent monoterpenes and monoterpenols and has no 1,8 cineole (oxide). Spanish Marjoram constituents are completely opposite, having a high content of 1,8 cineole and low levels of monoterpenes and monoterpenols. Sweet Marjoram enjoyed popularity as a common medicinal herb around the Mediterranean basin. A few drops can be diffused before bed, and a few drops can be added to a hot bath at the first signs of a cold. It is used in masculine, oriental, and herbal-spicy blends for perfumes and colognes. It is also a staple in insomnia blends.

- **Country of Origin:** France, Spain, South Africa
- **Extraction Method:** Steam Distillation
- **Plant Parts:** Flowers, leaves
- **Botanical Family:** Lamiaceae (Labiatae)
- **Latin Name:** Origanum marjorana
- **Chemical Families:** Monoterpenes, monoterpenols
- **Aroma:** Fresh, herbaceous, sweet, warm and radiant, woody
- **Note:** Middle

Precautions

- ☑ Non-toxic
- ☑ Non-irritating

Therapeutic Properties

Because Sweet Marjoram has high levels of monoterpenes and monoterpenals, it is most effective as tonifier, sedative and antiseptic. Where Spanish Marjoram, because of its high 1,8 cineole content, is more effective for respiratory congestion.

analgesic	antibacterial	antifungal
antispasmodic	cephalic	CNS sedative
digestive aid	vasodilator	warming
anti-infectious	regulates blood pressure	soothes muscles

Uses

- **Bones/Joints:** Aches, arthritis
- **Circulatory:** Circulatory disorders
- **Digestive:** Indigestion, constipation
- **Mental/Emotional:** Calms obsessive thinking, supports self-care, comforts and warms, calms the heart; insomnia, anxiety, nervous tension
- **Muscular/Joints:** Cramps, aches, rheumatism, sprains, headaches, spasms
- **Reproductive:** Cramps, menstrual problems, fluid retention.
- **Respiratory:** Decongestant, respiratory infections
- **Skin:** Bruises, burns, sores, cuts, sunburn

Application

Marjoram can be used topically, diffused, or inhaled. Add to a bath with some Lavender to aid in combating a migraine or insomnia attack. The cephalic property means the Marjoram not only soothes the nervous system but also clears the head. Use in a massage oil with a dilution of not more than 3% for all conditions.

Cautions

Marjoram is a benign and very beneficial herb, but the essential oil should be avoided during pregnancy.

Dilute before use; for external use only. Do not use on young children, and it may cause skin irritation in some individuals; a skin test is recommended prior to use. Contact with eyes should be avoided.

Essential Oil Datasheet

Mint (*Mentha longifolia*)

As one of twenty species in the Mentha family, Mentha Longifolia has been traditionally used for its medicinal properties. Also known as Horse Mint or Biblical Mint, it was mentioned in the Bible as one of the herbs and spices that were used as a tithe.

- **Country of Origin:** Native to Europe, Asia, and Africa
- **Extraction Method:** Steam Distillation
- **Plant Parts:** Aerial parts
- **Botanical Family:** Lamiaceae
- **Chemical Families:** Main constituent is piperitone
- **Aroma:** Fresh, minty scent that is milder than Peppermint
- **Blends Well With:** Eucalyptus, Lavender, Lemon, Rosemary, Basil, Benzoin
- **Note:** Top

Precautions

- ☑ Avoid during pregnancy
- ☑ May not be suitable to use on children
- ☑ Possible skin irritant

Therapeutic Properties

Mint may be used as an anti-asthmatic, carminative and stimulant. Its antiseptic, astringent and antibacterial properties make it useful for treating skin conditions. For muscular problems, it is also antispasmodic and antirheumatic.

antiseptic	anti-asthmatic	antispasmodic
carminative	stimulant	astringent
antirheumatic	antibacterial	

Uses

- **Digestive:** Indigestion, diarrhea, spasms, gas, reflux
- **Circulation:** Poor circulation
- **Muscular/Joints:** Headaches, arthritis, rheumatism
- **Mental/Emotional:** Insomnia
- Respiratory: Fever, bronchitis
- **Skin:** Inflammation, eczema, itching

Application

Mentha longifolia may be used in the same manner as the more readily available Spearmint and Peppermint essential oils. Mint can be diffused, inhaled or applied topically to the area. As a possible skin irritant, Mint is not recommended for use in baths.

Cautions

Mint is not suitable for use on children under 5 nor should it be used in sensitive areas. It should also be avoided during pregnancy.

Essential Oil Datasheet

Mustard Seed (*Brassica Nigra*)

Two different types of oil can be produced from mustard seeds: a vegetable oil and essential oil.

Mustard essential oil is different than the vegetable oil that is extracted by pressing the seeds, which produces a fatty oil used for cooking. Mustard essential oil is not recommended for general use in aromatherapy, due to its high level of toxicity. In the food industry, it is used in small quantities as a flavoring agent.

- **Country of Origin:** Europe and Asia
- **Extraction Method:** Seeds are ground and macerated in water, and then distilled
- **Plant Parts:** Seeds
- **Botanical Family:** Brassicaceae
- **Chemical Families:** Contains at least 92% allyl isothiocyanate
- **Aroma:** Hot, pungent, acrid scent
- **Blends Well With:** None
- **Note:** Middle

Precautions

- ☑ Considered to be a toxic essential oil
- ☑ Highly irritating to the skin and mucous membranes

Therapeutic Properties

The essential oil has emetic, diuretic, stimulant and aperitif properties, which are useful in treating digestive complaints, stomach upsets, and loss of appetite. For treating skin infections and wounds, it is antimicrobial and antiseptic. To remedy a fever, Mustard Seed oil can have a diaphoretic and febrifuge effect.

antimicrobial	antiseptic	diuretic
emetic	febrifuge	rubefacient
stimulant	diaphoretic	aperitif

Uses

- **Digestive:** Loss of appetite
- **Muscular/Joints:** Aches and pains, rheumatism
- **Respiratory:** Coughs, colds, chills
- **Nervous:** Neuralgia, numbness

Application

Due to its toxicity, Mustard Seed essential oil is not generally recommended for use in modern aromatherapy. However, a carrier oil made from Mustard Seed is considered safe to use. It is still sometimes used in India as a remedy for digestive and respiratory conditions, due to its warming and stimulating properties. It should never be inhaled or applied directly to the skin.

Cautions

Mustard Seed oil is extremely toxic and will irritate the skin and mucous membranes if topically applied or inhaled. It should be avoided during pregnancy.

Essential Oil Datasheet

Myrrh (*Commiphora myrrha*)

Ancients used Myrrh in religious ceremonies dating back thousands of years. This balsamic oil is known for calming and medicinal properties. Though it is classified as a shrub, Myrrh trees can grow up to 30 feet high. When the heartwood of the tree is pierced, a resin oozes out and hardens into reddish-brown droplets called "tears." Myrrh essential oil is renowned in aromatherapy circles for its ability to act as a servant oil. It aids in meditation and healing.

- **Country of Origin:** Ethiopia, South Africa
- **Extraction Method:** Steam Distillation
- **Plant Parts:** Resin/gum
- **Botanical Family:** Burseraceae
- **Chemical Families:** Sesqiterpenes, ketones
- **Aroma:** Balsamic, resinous, spicy, warm and radiant
- **Blends Well With:** Frankincense, Lavender, Patchouli, Sandalwood and Tea Tree
- **Note:** Base

Precautions

☑ Non-toxic
☑ Non-irritating

Therapeutic Properties

The high sesquiterpene content contributes to the anti-inflammatory and pain-relieving effects of Myrrh. Myrrh was highly prized amongst the Arabians because of its ability to treat skin conditions such as wrinkles, chapped and cracked skin. Like Clove Bud, Myrrh is used in a great number of oral hygiene products.

analgesic	anti-inflammatory	antibacterial
antifungal	astringent	cicatrisant
decongestant	skin healing	warming
anti-infectious	antiparasitic	antihyperthyroid

immune support	carminative	stomachic
anticatarrhal	expectorant	diaphoretic
vulnerary	local antiseptic	immune stimulant
circulatory stimulant	antispasmodic	

Uses

- **Bones/Joints:** Relieve toothaches, gum infections, gingivitis
- **Digestive:** Diarrhea, dysentery
- **Immune:** Antibacterial, antiviral
- **Mental/Emotional:** Offers emotional support, boosts energy
- **Muscular/Joints:** Arthritis
- **Reproductive:** Vaginal thrush
- **Respiratory:** Asthma, decongestant, bronchitis
- **Skin:** Stretch marks, skin conditions, eczema, chapped and cracked skin, wrinkles

Application

Diffuse or apply essential oil topically on location or use in massage oil. It also may be used as incense as many believe Myrrh essential oil promotes spiritual awareness and is uplifting.

Cautions

Myrrh can be toxic in high concentrations and should be avoided during pregnancy.

Essential Oil Datasheet

Myrtle (*Myrtus communis*)

Myrtle is used as an astringent, antiseptic, vulnerary, bactericidal, expectorant and decongestant.

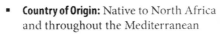

- **Country of Origin:** Native to North Africa and throughout the Mediterranean
- **Extraction Method:** Steam Distillation
- **Plant Parts:** Flower blossoms, leaves, twigs
- **Botanical Family:** Myrtaceae
- **Chemical Families:** Monoterpenes, monoterpenols, oxides
- **Aroma:** Balsamic, earthy, resinous, warm
- **Note:** Middle-Base
- **Strength of Aroma:** Medium
- **Blends Well With:** Bergamot, Clary Sage, Clove Bud, Hyssop, Eucalyptus, Ginger, Lavender, Peppermint, Rosemary, Spearmint, Thyme, and Tea Tree.

Precautions

- ☑ Can be irritating to the skin if oxidized
- ☑ Avoid use during pregnancy

Therapeutic Properties

Myrtle is effective for sore throats, coughs, and colds. It assists in easing a headache and reducing tension. Myrtle soothes the digestive tract and helps with stomach ailments, flatulence, and cramps associated with it.

anticatarrhal	anti-infectious	antispasmodic
carminative	cephalic	expectorant
tonic	stomachic	

Uses

- **Digestive:** good for diarrhea and dysentery.
- **Immune:** gentle and soothing for infections, immune support, flu, and colds.
- **Mental/Emotional:** great for the nervous system, uplifting, refreshing, helpful with self-destructive behavior, and to break addictions.
- **Muscular:** provides relief from arthritis and muscular pain.
- **Respiratory:** helpful for asthma, coughs, colds, congestion, excessive bronchial catarrh, and is useful for children's cough and chest complaints.
- **Skin/Hair:** useful for oily skin, infected skin, great to add to facial care products and toners, used for hemorrhoids.
- **Urinary/Genital:** can be used for bladder infections, cystitis, and aids in clearing congestion in the pelvic organs.

Application

Diffuse, apply topically or use in a humidifier. It is safe for children for chest complaints and coughs.

Cautions

Non-toxic, non-irritant and can be used by most. Safe for children. However, Myrtle essential oil can be possibly toxic in high concentrations, and should not be used during pregnancy.

Essential Oil Datasheet

Onycha (*Styrax benzoin*)

Benzoin (also referred to as Onycha in Bible times), was commonly used in the Middle East for incense and medicine. In the West, it is known for its use as a tincture of Friars Balsam for respiratory conditions.

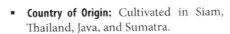

- **Country of Origin:** Cultivated in Siam, Thailand, Java, and Sumatra.
- **Extraction Method:** Resin absolute by steam distillation and/or extraction
- **Plant Parts:** Tree resin
- **Botanical Family:** Styracaceae
- **Chemical Families:** benzoate, styrene, benzyl alcohol, vanillin aldehyde, cinnamic acid
- **Aroma:** Warm, vanilla
- **Note:** Base

Precautions

☑ May cause skin irritation; always use a carrier oil or lotion when applying to skin

☑ Not recommended for use in baths

☑ Benzoin is safe to use during pregnancy after the second trimester and with children in a low dilution of 1% or less

Therapeutic Properties

While the absolutes and resinoids of Benzoin are frequently used as fixatives in perfumes and fragrances components in soaps, and cosmetics they are also frequently used in most food categories including alcoholic and soft drinks.

analgesic	antidepressant	anti-inflammatory
antioxidant	antiseptic	antispasmodic
astringent	antiviral	carminative
cephalic	cordial	deodorant

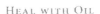

| diuretic | expectorant | sedative |
| tonic | vulnerary | |

Uses

- **Circulation:** treats arthritis, gout, poor circulation, rheumatism, muscle spasms, and fluid retention.
- **Digestive:** acts as a tonic for the liver and kidneys; good for irritable bowel syndrome, and prevents and relieves flatulence.
- **Immune:** one of the best-kept secrets for free radical scavenger, for inflammation and/or infection.
- **Mental/Emotional:** good for the nervous system, tension, and stress-related symptoms, depression, calming and soothing, counters anxiety, and insomnia.
- **Muscular/Joints:** treats rheumatic pain, back pain, and muscular aches and pains, and arthritis.
- **Respiration:** treats asthma, bronchitis, chills, colic, coughs, laryngitis, and issues with the mucus membrane.
- **Skin:** helps acne, cuts, eczema, irritated and inflamed skin, rashes, scar tissues and wounds that won't heal.

Application

Diffuse or apply on location. Approved by the FDA for use as a food additive (FA) and flavoring agent (FL).

Safety

Use in low dilution for therapeutic blends. Do not use in baths or massage oils.

Essential Oil Datasheet

Pine (*Pinus sylvestris*)

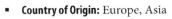

There are many varieties of Pine essential oil, although Pinus sylvestris (also known as Scotch Pine) is considered to be the safest for use in aromatherapy. Its fresh, forest-like aroma is refreshing and cleansing, particularly for respiratory ailments.

- **Country of Origin:** Europe, Asia
- **Extraction Method:** Dry Distillation
- **Plant Parts:** Needles
- **Botanical Family:** Pinaceae
- **Chemical Families:** Monoterpene hydrocarbons (50-90%)
- **Aroma:** Strong, fresh, woody, balsamic scent
- **Blends Well With:** Cedarwood, Rosemary, Tea Tree, Lavender, Juniper, Eucalyptus, Lemon
- **Note:** Middle

Precautions

- ☑ Generally non-toxic, but should be used in moderation
- ☑ May irritate the skin and mucous membranes
- ☑ Avoid using on sensitive skin

Therapeutic Properties

Pine is a popular cleansing agent, due to its antimicrobial, antiseptic, antiviral, bactericidal, deodorant, insecticidal and vermifuge properties. It is an energizing oil with diuretic, hypertensive, restorative, rubefacient and stimulant effects on the body. Pine is also an antirheumatic, cholagogue and expectorant.

antimicrobial	antirheumatic	antiseptic
antiviral	bactericidal	cholagogue
deodorant	diuretic	expectorant
hypertensive	insecticidal	restorative
rubefacient	stimulant	vermifuge

Uses

- **Circulatory:** Poor circulation
- **Genito-Urinary:** Cystitis, urinary infections
- **Mental/Emotional:** Stress, mental fatigue
- **Muscular/Joints:** Arthritis, gout, aches, and pains, rheumatism
- **Respiratory:** Asthma, bronchitis, catarrh, coughs, tonsillitis, sinusitis, colds, flu
- **Nervous:** Fatigue, nervous exhaustion, neuralgia
- **Skin:** Cuts, sores, lice

Application

For respiratory conditions, use Pine in an inhalation to relieve catarrh and congestion. A low dosage should be used in order to prevent irritation of the mucous membranes. Pine may also be diffused or applied topically. The fresh, cleansing aroma of Pine makes it a popular oil for diffusion – particularly around Christmas time.

Cautions

Pine is generally non-toxic but has the potential to irritate the skin and mucous membranes. For this reason, it is best to only use this oil in moderation and avoid using on sensitive skin.

Essential Oil Datasheet

Rose of Isaiah (*Narcissus tazetta*)

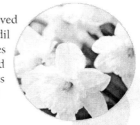

Despite its name, this essential oil is not derived from a rose at all. Belonging to the daffodil family, Narcissus tazetta is sometimes referred to as French Daffodil. It is mentioned in the Bible's Book of Isaiah, which translates the name from Hebrew into 'Rose of Isaiah.'

- **Country of Origin:** Israel, Jordan
- **Extraction Method:** Enfleurage or solvent extraction
- **Plant Parts:** Flowers
- **Botanical Family:** Amaryllidaceae
- **Chemical Families:** Main component is trans-ocimene (65%)
- **Aroma:** Sweet, floral, fruity
- **Blends Well With:** Rose, Sandalwood, Jasmine, Neroli, Ylang Ylang
- **Note:** Middle

Precautions

- ☑ Avoid during pregnancy
- ☑ May cause headaches, skin rashes, dizziness, convulsions, vomiting, paralysis or even death

Therapeutic Properties

Narcissus tazetta is analgesic, anti-inflammatory and antispasmodic, which makes it useful for treating muscular-related ailments. Its antibacterial, demulcent and antifungal properties help with skin conditions and infections. It is also an emetic, narcotic, sedative, aphrodisiac and diuretic.

emetic	demulcent	analgesic
anti-inflammatory	antispasmodic	narcotic
sedative	aphrodisiac	diuretic
antibacterial	antifungal	insecticidal

Uses

- **Immune:** Tumors, bacterial infections
- **Mental/Emotional:** Stress, tension, anxiety
- **Muscular/Joints:** Headaches
- **Nervous:** Epilepsy, hysteria
- **Skin:** Abscesses, boils, baldness, fungal infections

Application

Narcissus oils are not recommended for therapeutic use in modern aromatherapy, but may be used as perfume.

Cautions

Rose of Isaiah should be avoided during pregnancy and is not generally recommended for therapeutic use in aromatherapy. Side effects may include headaches, rashes, dizziness, seizures, vomiting, paralysis, or – in extreme cases – even death.

Essential Oil Datasheet

Rose of Sharon (*Cistus labdanum or Cistus ladanifer*)

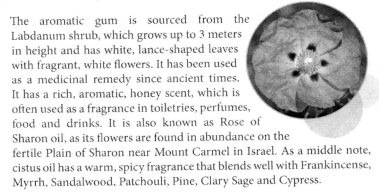

The aromatic gum is sourced from the Labdanum shrub, which grows up to 3 meters in height and has white, lance-shaped leaves with fragrant, white flowers. It has been used as a medicinal remedy since ancient times. It has a rich, aromatic, honey scent, which is often used as a fragrance in toiletries, perfumes, food and drinks. It is also known as Rose of Sharon oil, as its flowers are found in abundance on the fertile Plain of Sharon near Mount Carmel in Israel. As a middle note, cistus oil has a warm, spicy fragrance that blends well with Frankincense, Myrrh, Sandalwood, Patchouli, Pine, Clary Sage and Cypress.

- **Country of Origin:** France, Spain, Israel
- **Extraction Method:** Solvent Extraction or Steam Distillation
- **Plant Parts:** Gum or leaves/twigs
- **Botanical Family:** Cistaceae
- **Chemical Families:** Contains over 170 pinenes
- **Aroma:** Rich, warm, spicy, honey-citrus scent
- **Blends Well With:** Frankincense, Myrrh, Sandalwood, Patchouli, Pine, Clary Sage, Cypress and Vetiver
- **Note:** Middle

Precautions

☑ Avoid during pregnancy

Therapeutic Properties

Cistus Labdanum oil is useful for treating infectious conditions, as it has antiviral, antibacterial, antimicrobial, antiseptic, astringent and anti-infectious properties. It is also an anti-inflammatory, antihemorrhagic, immune stimulant, antitussive, expectorant, tonic and emmenagogue oil. It supports the sympathetic nervous system and is an immune stimulant. Rose of Sharon can be useful for bronchitis, respiratory infections, coughs, rhinitis, urinary tract infections, wounds, wrinkles, hemorrhages, arthritis, and is known for elevating the emotions and calming the nerves. It helps reduce inflammation and is a neurotonic for the sympathetic nervous system.

anti-infectious	antiviral	antibacterial
antihemorrhagic	anti-inflammatory	immune stimulant
antimicrobial	antiseptic	antitussive
astringent	balsamic	emmenagogue
expectorant	tonic	

Uses

- **Immune:** Strengthens and stimulates the immune system
- **Mental/Emotional:** Elevates the emotions and calms the nerves; research has been done on its effects on the regeneration of cells.
- **Muscular/Joints:** Eases arthritic pain
- **Genito-Urinary:** Can be used to fight urinary tract infections
- **Respiratory:** Helps to treat bronchitis, respiratory infections, colds, coughs and rhinitis
- **Nervous:** Supports the sympathetic nervous system
- **Skin:** Can be used as a treatment for cuts, wounds and wrinkles. It helps to reduce hemorrhage and inflammation.

Application

Cistus oil may be diffused, inhaled, used in baths or applied (2-4 drops) directly to the affected area.

Cautions

Labdanum essential oil is generally non-toxic and non-sensitizing. Avoid use during pregnancy.

Essential Oil Datasheet

Rue (*Ruta graveolens*)

Although not commonly used in modern aromatherapy, Rue was traditionally used as an herbal remedy by ancient civilizations. It was thought to ward off evil and help with nervous disorders, digestive complaints, and venomous bites.

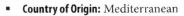

- **Country of Origin:** Mediterranean
- **Extraction Method:** Steam Distillation
- **Plant Parts:** Leaves
- **Botanical Family:** Rutaceae
- **Chemical Families:** Methyl nonyl ketone is the primary constituent
- **Aroma:** Sharp, herbaceous, fruity scent
- **Blends Well With:** Chamomile, Myrrh, Bay, Fennel, Frankincense, Thyme, Benzoin
- **Note:** Top

Precautions

- ☑ Avoid during pregnancy
- ☑ Irritant to the skin and mucous membranes
- ☑ Highly toxic
- ☑ Not recommended for general use in aromatherapy

Therapeutic Properties

Rue is a strengthening oil, due to its stimulant, tonic, antitoxic and nervine properties. It is also an antitussive, antiseptic, antispasmodic, diuretic, emmenagogue, insecticidal, rubefacient and vermifuge oil.

antitoxic	antitussive	antiseptic
antispasmodic	diuretic	emmenagogue
insecticidal	nervine	rubefacient
stimulant	tonic	vermifuge

Uses

- **Digestive:** Colic, poor digestion, loss of appetite, food poisoning
- **Menstrual:** Amenorrhea, dysmenorrhea
- **Immune:** Bacterial infections
- **Mental/Emotional:** Stress, insomnia
- **Muscular/Joints:** Arthritis, rheumatism, aches, and pains
- **Nervous:** Convulsions
- **Skin:** Fungal skin conditions, insect bites, stings

Application

Rue essential oil is not recommended for use in general aromatherapy.

Cautions

Rue should be avoided during pregnancy, and is not generally recommended for use in modern aromatherapy. The oil is highly toxic and will irritate the skin and mucous membranes.

Essential Oil Datasheet

Saffron (*Crocus sativa*)

Crocus sativus or Saffron essential oil is known as one of the most expensive spices because of the stigmas of the plant that are handpicked to make the spice. It has a herbaceous, warm, woodsy aroma. One of the earliest historical references mentioning Saffron comes out of ancient Egypt where the stigmas were used in perfumes, hair and fabric dyes, as well as culinary purposes and as a drug.

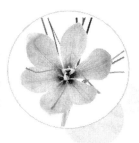

- **Country of Origin:** Iran, India
- **Extraction Method:** Steam Distillation
- **Plant Parts:** Flowers
- **Botanical Family:** Iridaceae
- **Chemical Families:** Terpenes
- **Aroma:** Herbaceous, warm, woodsy, hay-like odor
- **Blends Well:** Saffron Absolute essential oil blends well with most exotic florals
- **Note:** Middle

Precautions

- ☑ Avoid use during pregnancy
- ☑ Do not use on children
- ☑ Do not use in eyes or near mucous membranes
- ☑ Can irritate skin; use at low dilution

Therapeutic Properties

antibacterial	sedative	expectorant
aphrodisiac	diaphoretic	anti-aging
antioxidant	pain reliever	anti-inflammatory
good for digestion	stimulants appetite	antidepressant
antiviral	hypotensive	reduces cholesterol
strengthens cardio	anti-cancer	memory-enhancing

Uses

- **Circulatory:** The presence of crocetin makes it helpful in reducing the blood cholesterol levels and triglycerides and strengthening the heart. It is said to have active ingredients that lower blood pressure.

- **Digestion:** Saffron is said to help in digestion and increases appetite. It is also used to get relief from renal colic and stomach aches.

- **Immune:** It has compounds that increase antibacterial and antiviral physiological activity in the body. Researches have demonstrated anti-cancer and antioxidant activities of Saffron extracts.

- **Mental/Emotional:** Research has shown it is memory-enhancing and supports the nervous system. Folkloric uses of Saffron include its use as a sedative. Helps with depression and insomnia. It is said to be beneficial in treating alcoholism. Studies have shown it to help with mild to moderate Alzheimer's disease. Other uses include depression, improving moods and PMS.

- **Muscular:** A few drops of Saffron essential oil may be mixed with half a teaspoon of almond oil and rubbed directly into the joints. It is also is a potent antioxidant that relieves both pain and inflammation.

- **Respiratory:** Strengthens the lungs; good for the common cold; expectorant; eases asthma. Good for menstrual problems.

- **Reproductive:** Used as an aphrodisiac and diaphoretic. Good for menstrual cramps, PMS, and kidney stones.

- **Skin/Hair:** Used for skin lightening, anti-aging creams, and other beauty products. Good for sore gums.

Application

Use at low dilutions.

Cautions

It contains chemicals known as Safranal and is restricted by IFRA to 0.005% in perfumes. Use with caution in soaps and perfumes.

Essential Oil Datasheet

Sandalwood (*Santalum album*)

Alpha-santalol gives Sandalwood much of its characteristic scent. Research shows the combination of alpha and beta santalol contributes to the sedative and anti-infectious effects of Sandalwood oil. The Sandalwood tree is cut down, and its wood is distilled. This presents some ecological issues, and the oil should be used with respect. Some studies show Sandalwood could be an effective preventative agent in skin cancer.

- **Country of Origin:** Hawaii, India, Australia
- **Extraction Method:** Steam Distillation
- **Plant Parts:** Trunks
- **Botanical Family:** Santalaceae
- **Chemical Families:** Sesquiterpenes, sesquiterpenols
- **Aroma:** Balsamic, earthy, sweet, warm, radiant, woody
- **Note:** Base

Precautions

☑ In rare cases, it may cause skin sensitization and should be used topically at 2% dilution

☑ Avoid during pregnancy

Therapeutic Properties

Sandalwood supports meditation and quiets mental activity. Reduces irritation and aggressive behavior. Provides protection and encourages acceptance emotionally. Works well in creams for skin conditions and is great for sore throats and cold sores.

anti-inflammatory	antifungal	antispasmodic
antiviral	astringent	sedative
cooling	decongestant	skin healing
wound healing (burns)		

Uses

- **Circulation:** good for circulatory complaints such as rheumatism and arthritis.
- **Mental/Emotional:** tonic for the nervous system serves to quiet the mind and compulsive behavior. Sedative-like qualities.
- **Respiratory:** used for sinus congestion, colds, and coughs.
- **Skin:** good for skin care and is very calming to irritated, dry, scaly patches. Used for skin cancer. Heals wounds and burns.

Application

Sandalwood can be diffused and applied to the skin with a carrier oil.

Cautions

There are no known risks from using Sandalwood oil. However, it is recommended to always dilute before applying to the skin. Non-toxic; however, if oxidized it may cause skin irritation or sensitization. Avoid during pregnancy.

Essential Oil Datasheet

Spikenard (*Nardostachys jatamansi*)

Spikenard is used by aromatherapists for rashes, wrinkles, cuts, insomnia, migraines, and wounds. It brings peaceful tranquility.

- **Country of Origin:** India and Nepal
- **Extraction Method:** Steam Distillation
- **Plant Parts:** Root
- **Botanical Family:** Valerianaceae
- **Chemical Families:** Sesquiterpenes, sesquiterpenols
- **Aroma:** Earthy, exotic, sensual, resinous, woodsy
- **Note:** Base

Precautions

☑ Avoid during pregnancy

Therapeutic Properties

This oil's therapeutic properties are anti-inflammatory, antifungal, antispasmodic, sedative and tonic.

anti-inflammatory	sedative	grounding
antifungal	antispasmodic	tonic
antibacterial	deodorant	relaxing

Uses

- **Mental/Emotional:** Great for quieting the mind, calming the heart, stabilizing the mind and settling the emotions. Used for insomnia, anxiety, and other emotional disorders.
- **Skin/Hair:** useful for athlete's foot and other fungal skin infections. Works great in skin care products for the mature and aging skin. Perfumes the hair. Anti-inflammatory benefits work on wounds for faster healing and scarring tissue.
- **Circulation:** recent studies show it has been used successfully to deal with tachycardia.

Application

Can be inhaled from the bottle, applied to the abdomen, or on location for soothing and calming.

Cautions

Non-toxic, non-irritant and can be used by most.

Essential Oil Datasheet

Terebinth (*Pistacia terebinthus*)

As its botanical name suggests, Terebinth oil belongs to the same family as the pistachio. It is a flowering plant, commonly known as Indian Turpentine or turpentine tree, which is the earliest known source of turpentine. It does not produce common turpentine, which is derived from pine trees.

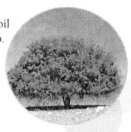

- **Country of Origin:** Mediterranean
- **Extraction Method:** Hydro-Distillation
- **Plant Parts:** Aerial parts
- **Botanical Family:** Anacardiaceae
- **Chemical Families:** Pinene, terpinene, limonene
- **Aroma:** Warm, balsamic scent
- **Blends Well With:** Benzoin, Cypress, Eucalyptus
- **Note:** Middle

Precautions

- Avoid in pregnancy
- May cause skin irritation or sensitization
- May damage the kidneys in large doses

Therapeutic Properties

Terebinth is a versatile plant, offering many therapeutic properties that have been recognized by herbalists for thousands of years. It is analgesic, antirheumatic and antispasmodic, which helps with muscular and joint problems. For infections and respiratory disorders, it offers antimicrobial, antiseptic, expectorant and tonic properties. It is also used as an aphrodisiac, stimulant, tonic, vermifuge and diuretic.

analgesic	antimicrobial	antirheumatic
antiseptic	antispasmodic	balsamic
diuretic	expectorant	rubefacient
stimulant	tonic	vermifuge
aphrodisiac		

Uses

- **Digestive:** Indigestion, tapeworm
- **Genito-Urinary:** Urethritis, cystitis
- **Circulatory:** Poor circulation
- **Muscular/Joints:** Rheumatism, arthritis, aches and pains, gout, stiffness
- **Respiratory:** Excess phlegm, bronchitis, colds
- **Nervous:** Neuralgia
- **Skin:** Boils, sores, toothache, dermatitis, ringworm, wounds, fleas, cuts

Application

Terebinth may be diffused or applied topically in a low dilution. Alternatively, it may be inhaled to treat respiratory conditions. As a possible irritant, it is not recommended for use in baths, and should always be used in low dilutions.

Cautions

Terebinth oil should not be used in pregnancy. It may also cause skin irritation or sensitization, so is best avoided by those with sensitive skin. In large doses, it can damage the kidneys.

Essential Oil Datasheet

Wormwood (Artemisia judaica)

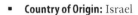

There are many varieties of Wormwood within the Artemisia family. Artemisia judaica or Judean Wormwood is mentioned in the Bible's Old Testament. Described as a poison, it was also used as a metaphor for sadness.

- **Country of Origin:** Israel
- **Extraction Method:** Steam Distillation
- **Plant Parts:** Aerial parts
- **Botanical Family:** Asteraceae
- **Chemical Families:** Main components are piperitone (45%) and trans-ethyl cinnamate (20.8%)
- **Aroma:** Spicy, warm, bitter
- **Blends Well With:** Lavender, Jasmine, Orange
- **Note:** Top

Precautions

- ☑ Avoid during pregnancy
- ☑ Highly toxic – may cause kidney irritation, gastro-enteritis, stupors, seizures, vision problems or even death
- ☑ Not recommended for general use in aromatherapy

Therapeutic Properties

Wormwood has analgesic, anti-inflammatory and antispasmodic properties, which can help with muscular aches and pains. It is also thought to be stomachic, expectorant, diaphoretic, insecticide, antimicrobial, antioxidant, tonic, stimulant and vermifuge.

stomachic	expectorant	analgesic
diaphoretic	antispasmodic	insecticide
anti-inflammatory	antimicrobial	antioxidant
tonic	stimulant	vermifuge

Uses

- **Digestive:** Intestinal parasites, stomach aches, indigestion
- **Menstrual:** Amenorrhea, dysmenorrhea
- **Muscular/Joints:** Muscular aches and pains

Application

Wormwood essential oil is not suitable for diffusion, inhalation or applying to the skin. Some varieties of Wormwood essential oil are available to purchase, but should only be used at your own risk.

Cautions

Wormwood essential oil is not generally recommended for therapeutic use in modern aromatherapy. It should certainly be avoided in pregnancy. The oil is highly toxic, to the extent that it may have fatal consequences. Other known side effects may include kidney damage, gastro-enteritis, stupors, seizures and vision problems.

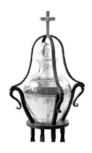

Essential Oil Storage AND SAFETY

Because essential oils contain no fatty acids, they are not susceptible to rancidity like vegetable oils – but you will want to protect them from the degenerative effects of heat, light and air. Store them in tightly sealed, dark glass bottles away from any heat source. Properly stored oils can maintain their quality for years.

ESSENTIAL OIL STORAGE TIPS

- Keep oils tightly closed and out of reach of children.
- Always read and follow all label warnings and cautions.
- Do not purchase essential oils with rubber glass dropper tops. Essential oils are highly concentrated and will turn the rubber to gum, thus ruining the oil.
- Make note of when the bottle of essential oil was opened and its shelf life.
- Many essential oils will remove the furniture's finish. Use care when handling open bottles.
- Store essential oil in a dark place away from light or heat.
- Be selective of where you purchase your essential oils. The quality of essential oil varies widely from company to company. Additionally, some companies may falsely claim their oils are undiluted and pure when they are not.

ESSENTIAL OIL SAFETY USAGE

In general, essential oils are safe to use for aromatherapy and therapeutic purposes. Nonetheless, safety must be exercised due to their potency and high concentration. Please read and follow these guidelines to obtain the maximum effectiveness and benefits.

- Avoid sunbathing, tanning booths, or a using a sauna immediately after using essential oils.

- Be careful to avoid getting essential oils in the eyes. If you do splash a drop or two of essential oil in the eyes, use a small amount of Olive oil (or another carrier oil) to dilute the essential oil and absorb with a washcloth. If serious, seek medical attention immediately.

- Take extra precaution when using oils with children. Never use undiluted essential oils on babies and always store your essential oils out of the reach of children.

- Never take essential oils internally, unless advised by your medical practitioner or another qualified health professional.

- If a dangerous quantity of essential oil has been ingested immediately, drink Olive oil and induce vomiting. The Olive oil will help in slowing down its absorption and dilute the essential oil. Do not drink water – this will speed up the absorption of the essential oil.

- Most essential oils should be diluted before applying topically. Pay attention to safety guidelines – certain essential oils such as Cinnamon may cause skin irritation for those with sensitive skin. If you experience slight redness or itchiness, put Olive oil (or any carrier oil) on the affected area and cover with a soft cloth. The Olive oil acts as an absorbent fat and binds to the oil, diluting its strength and allowing it to be immediately removed. Aloe Vera gel also works well as an alternative to Olive oil. Never use water to dilute essential oil – this will cause it to spread and enlarge the affected area.

Redness or irritation may last 20 minutes to an hour.

- Never use oils undiluted on your skin. Always dilute with a carrier oil. If redness, burning, itching or irritation occurs, stop using oil immediately. Be sure to wash hands after handling pure, undiluted essential oils.
- For sensitive skin, if irritation occurs, discontinue use of such oil.
- If you are pregnant, lactating, suffer from epilepsy or high blood pressure, have cancer, liver damage, or another medical condition, use essential oils under the care and supervision of a qualified aromatherapist or medical practitioner.
- If taking prescription drugs, check for interaction between medicine and essential oils (if any) to avoid interference with certain prescription medications.
- To prevent contact sensitization (redness or irritation of skin due to repeated use of same individual oil) rotate and use different oils.

ESSENTIAL OIL PRECAUTIONS

Do Not Use These Oils Anytime: Calamus, Mustard, and Rue

Oils That May Be Mucous Membrane Irritants: Cassia, Cinnamon

Oils Not Recommended For Use in Bath: Benzoin, Cassia, Cinnamon, Marjoram, and Pine

Oils Not Recommended For Children Under 5 Years: Cedarwood (*Cedrus atlantica*), Fennel, Hyssop, and Marjoram

Oils to Avoid With Epilepsy: Fennel, Hyssop, and Wormwood

Oils to Avoid With Low Blood Pressure: Marjoram

Oils Not Recommended For Long-Term Use (more than 10 days in a row): Fennel and Marjoram

Oils to Avoid During Various Trimesters of Pregnancy: Anise, Bay Laurel, Cistus, Cedarwood, Cinnamon, Cumin, Cypress, Fennel, Frankincense, Hyssop, Marjoram, and Myrrh

Oils Not Recommended For Sensitive Skin (or should be diluted): Anise, Bay Laurel, Fennel, Pine and Spruce

Oils That May Be Phototoxic or Cause Sun Sensitivity: Cumin

Oils That May Be Potentially Toxic: Wormwood

Oils Considered Very Toxic: Calamus, Mustard, and Rue

Oils to Avoid With History of Estrogen-Dependent Cancer: Cypress, Fennel, Myrrh, and Pine (prostate cancer)

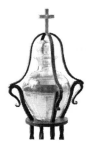

Glossary
OF TERMS

Abortifacient
A substance or agent that can induce abortion.

Absorption Rate
The rate at which an essential oil or carrier oil penetrates the skin over a given period of time (can be subjective).

Absolute
A concentrated, highly aromatic, oily mixture extracted from plants by means of solvent extraction techniques producing a waxy mass called concrete. The lower

molecular weight, fragrant compounds are extracted from the concrete into ethanol. When the ethanol evaporates, the absolute is left behind.

Adulterate
To make impure by adding extraneous, improper, or inferior ingredients.

Allergy
A hypersensitivity to certain substances such as pollens, foods, or microorganisms which cause an overreaction of the immune system with symptoms such as a skin rash, swelling of mucous membranes, sneezing or wheezing, or other abnormal conditions.

Alterative
A substance that gradually nourishes and improves the system.

Analgesic
An agent that relieves pain by acting upon the peripheral and central nervous systems.

Anaphrodisiac
The decline or absence of sexual desire.

Anesthetic
An agent that produces anesthesia by paralyzing sensory nerve endings (or partial loss of sensation) at the site of application.

Anodyne
An agent that relieves pain.

Anthelmintic

An agent that destroys or causes the expulsion of parasitic intestinal worms.

Anti-allergenic

A substance capable of preventing an allergic reaction.

Anti-anxiety

An agent capable of preventing or reducing anxiety.

Anti-arthritic

An agent that alleviates arthritis by providing therapy to relieve the symptoms of joint inflammation.

Anti-asthmatic

An agent that provides relief from asthma or halts an asthmatic attack.

Antibacterial

An agent capable of destroying or inhibiting the growth or reproduction of bacteria.

Anticoagulant

A substance that inhibits the clotting of blood by blocking the action of clotting factors or platelets.

Anticonvulsant

An agent that helps prevents or reduces the severity of epileptic or other convulsive seizures.

Antidepressant

A substance or an agent used to alleviate mood disorders such as depression and anxiety and/or prevent clinical depression.

Antidontalgic
A substance that has the ability to relieve a toothache.

Anti-emetic
An agent that prevents or alleviates nausea and vomiting.

Antifungal
A substance used to treat fungal infections such as athlete's foot, ringworm, candidiasis (thrush), and serious infections such as cryptococcal meningitis.

Antihistamine
A compound that inhibits the production of histamine, primarily used in the treatment of allergies and colds.

Antihemorrhagic
A substance that prevents or stops bleeding.

Anti-infectious
An agent capable of stopping the colonization of a microscopic organism such as a virus or bacteria.

Anti-inflammatory
A substance that prevents or reduces certain types of inflammation such as swelling, tenderness, fever, and pain.

Antimicrobial
An agent capable of destroying or inhibiting the growth of microorganisms.

Antineuralgic
An agent that relieves neuralgia, an intense burning or stabbing pain caused by irritation of or damage to a nerve caused by disease, inflammation, or infection.

Antioxidant
A substance that retards or inhibits oxidation.

Antiparasitic
An agent that destroys and inhibits the growth of parasites.

Antiphlogistic
A substance that functions to relieve inflammation and fever.

Antipruritic
An agent that prevents or relieves itching.

Antipyretic
An agent that reduces fever.

Antirheumatic
An agent that suppresses the manifestation of rheumatic disease and has the capability of delaying the progression of the disease process in inflammatory arthritis; it provides relief of the symptoms of any painful or immobilizing disorder of the musculoskeletal system.

Antisclerotic
An agent that helps to prevent hardening of arteries or is affected with sclerosis.

Antiseborrheic
An agent applied to the skin to control seborrhea or the excessive oily secretion of sebum in the sweat glands.

Antiscorbutic
Refers to an agent that cures or prevents scurvy.

Antiseptic
Refers to a substance capable of preventing infection by inhibiting the growth and reproduction of microorganisms.

Antispasmodic
An agent that relieves or prevents spasms, particularly of smooth muscle.

Antisudorific
A substance that is capable of inhibiting the secretion of sweat.

Antitoxic
An agent that neutralizes the action of a toxin or poison.

Antitussive
A substance that suppresses the body's urge to cough.

Antivenomous
An antitoxin active against the venom of a snake, spider, or other venomous animal or insect.

Antiviral
An agent or substance capable of destroying a virus and/or inhibits it from spreading and reproducing.

Aperient
A substance that gently stimulates the evacuation of the bowels and works as a mild laxative.

Aphrodisiac
A substance that arouses or intensifies sexual desire and function.

Aromatherapy
The art and science of using essential oils to heal common ailments and complaints. Therapy with aroma can be particularly helpful with stress or emotionally triggered problems such as insomnia and headaches. The term "aromatherapy" was coined by a French chemist, R.M. Gattefosse.

Astringent
A substance that draws together or constricts body tissues and that is effective in stopping the flow of blood or other secretions.

Attar (Otto)
From the ancient Persian word "to smell sweet." Attar or Otto refers to essential oil obtained by distillation and, in particular, that of the Bulgarian Rose, an extremely precious perfumery material.

Ayurvedic
The ancient Hindu art of medicine and of prolonging life.

Balsam
A water soluble, semi-solid or viscous resinous exudates similar to that of gum.

Balsamic
A soothing substance that has the qualities of balsam.

Bechic
An agent that relieves coughing.

Botanical Name
A scientific name in Latin that conforms to the International Code of Botanical Nomenclature (ICBN) and is of a certain species of plant that clearly distinguishes it from other plants that share the same common name. The purpose of a formal name is to have a single name that is accepted and used worldwide for a particular plant or plant group.

Calming
A substance that causes a sense of serenity, tranquility and/or peace.

Calmative
An agent that has relaxing or sedating properties.

Carminative
An agent that induces the expulsion of gas from the stomach or intestines settles the digestive system and relieves flatulence.

Carrier Oil
A vegetable fatty oil used to dilute essential oils for the purpose of application to the skin or massage.

Cephalic
A substance that clears the mind.

Chemotypes
The same botanical species occurring in other forms due to different growth conditions.

Cholagogue
An agent that promotes the discharge of bile from the system, purging it downward.

Cicatrisant
An agent that promotes the formation of scar tissue.

Circulatory Stimulant
A substance that temporarily increases circulation and invigorates the circulatory system.

CO2 Extracts
Oils that are extracted by the carbon dioxide method are commonly referred to as CO2 Extracts or CO2s for short. Essential oils processed by this method are considered superior in that none of the constituents have been harmed by heat, have a closer aroma to the natural source and are generally thicker oils.

Cold-pressed
Refers to a method of extraction where no external heat is applied during the process.

Common Name
The everyday name used for a plant. Names such as Frankincense, Myrrh, or Mint may refer to more than one species, yet go by the same name. It is necessary to know its botanical name for clarity.

Concrete
A waxy concentrate semi-solid essential oil extract, made from plant material that is used to make an absolute.

Cooling
A substance that offers relief from the heat and has a calming effect.

Cytotoxic
An agent that is toxic to all cells.

Decoction
An herbal preparation made by boiling the plant material and reducing into a concentration.

Decongestant
An agent that treats sinus congestion by reducing swelling.

Demulcent
An agent that soothes irritated mucous membranes and relieves pain and inflammation.

Depurative
A substance that is purgative or used for purifying.

Dermatitis
Inflammation of the skin.

Detoxifier
A substance that helps to detoxify and remove impurities from the blood and body.

Diaphoretic
An agent that promotes perspiration.

Diffuser
A device used to disperse the aromatic molecules of essential oils into the air.

Distillation
A method of extraction employed in the manufacture of essential oils.

Diuretic
A substance that increases the flow of urine, thus removing water from the body.

Emetic
A substance that induces vomiting.

Emmenagogue
A substance that is used to stimulate blood flow to the pelvic area and uterus; some stimulate menstruation.

Essential Fatty Acids (EFA)
These are the fatty acids that are necessary for our body to function properly, but cannot produce on its own. When the body is deprived of these nutrients, skin conditions such as eczema or psoriasis may appear.

Essential Oil
An aromatic, volatile liquid consisting of odorous principles from plant extracts.

Expectorant
An agent that promotes the secretion or expulsion of phlegm, mucus, or other matter from the respiratory passages.

Expression
An extraction method where plant materials are pressed to obtain the essential oil.

Exudates
A natural substance secreted by plants – can be spontaneous or after damage to the plant.

Febrifuge
An agent that reduces fever.

Fixative
A natural or synthetic substance used to slow down the evaporation of volatile components in a perfume and improve stability when added to more volatile components.

Fixed Oils
Vegetable oils obtained from plants that are fatty and non-volatile.

Fractionated Oil
A process in which oils are re-distilled, either to have terpenes or other substances removed.

Fungicide
A substance that destroys or inhibits the growth of fungi.

Galactagogue
An agent that induces milk secretion.

Germicidal
An agent that kills germs, especially pathogenic microorganisms, and acts as a disinfectant.

Hemostatic
An agent that stops bleeding or hemorrhaging.

Hepatoxic
An agent that has a toxic or harmful effect on the liver.

Hydro-Distillation

A method of extracting essential oils in which steam at atmospheric pressure is passed through the plant material from the top of the extraction chamber, resulting in oils that retain the original aroma of the plant and is less harsh than steam distillation.

Hydrosol (Floral Water)

The water resulting from the distillation of essential oils, which still contains some of the properties of the plant material from the extraction process.

Hypertension

Arterial disease in which chronic high blood pressure is the primary symptom.

Hypertensive

An agent that raises blood pressure.

Hypotension

Abnormally low blood pressure.

Immuno-stimulant

An agent that stimulates an immune response.

Immune Support

An agent that supports the immune system and assists in the resistance to infection by a specific pathogen.

Infused Oil

Oil produced by steeping the macerated botanical material in liquid until it has taken on some of the plant material's properties.

Infusion
The process of making an herbal remedy by steeping plant material in water to extract its soluble principles.

Lipolytic
The chemical reaction of lipolysis, which is the disintegration of fats.

Lymphatic Support
Offers support to a lymph, a lymph vessel, or a lymph node.

Macerate
To make soft by soaking or steeping in a liquid.

Massage Therapy
The manipulation of soft tissue of the body to enhance health and is known to affect the circulation of blood and the flow of blood and lymph, reduce muscular tension or flaccidity, affect the nervous system through stimulation or <u>sedation</u>, and enhance tissue healing.

Microbe
Minute living organism, such as pathogenic bacteria and viruses, that cause disease.

Mucilage
A gummy substance containing demulcent gelatinous constituents obtained from certain plants.

Mucolytic
Denotes an enzyme that breaks down mucus.

Nervine

An agent that has a soothing or calming effect upon the nerves.

Neurotoxin

A substance that is poisonous or destructive to nerve tissue.

Oleoresin

Natural resinous exudation from plants or aromatic liquid extracted from botanical material.

Olfaction

Refers to the sense of smell.

Olfactory Bulb

The bulb-like distal end of the olfactory lobe center where the processing of smell is started and is then passed to other areas of the brain.

Oxidation

The process of the addition of oxygen to an organic molecule, or the removal of electrons or hydrogen from the molecule.

Pathogenic

An agent that causes disease.

Pharmacology

The science that deals with the origin, nature, chemistry, effects, and uses of drugs.

Pheromone

A substance released by an animal that serves to influence the physiology or behavior of other members of the same species, such as chemical messenger sent between two people.

Phytohormones
Plant substances mimicking the actions of human hormones. Plant hormones in the plant control or regulate germination, growth, metabolism, or other physiological activities.

Phytotherapy
The use of natural plant extracts for medicinal purposes as in the treatment of disease.

Pomade
Perfumed fat obtained from the effleurage extraction method.

Prophylactic
An act of preventing disease or infection.

Resin
A natural substance exuded from trees; prepared resins are oleoresins from which the essential oil has been removed.

Resinoids
Perfumed material extracted from natural resinous material by solvent extraction.

Resolvent
A substance that reduces inflammation or swelling.

Rubefacient
A substance that irritates the skin, causing redness.

Sedative

An agent that has a soothing, calming, or tranquilizing effect upon the body, reducing or relieving anxiety, stress, irritability, or excitement.

Shelf Life

The amount of time a carrier or base oil will remain fresh before oxidizing and become rancid.

Soporific

A substance that produces deep sleep.

Stomachic

A substance that aids in digestion in the stomach and improves appetite.

Styptic

An agent that contracts the tissues or blood vessels; used particularly to control hemorrhaging and stop external bleeding.

Sudorific

An agent that causes or increases sweat.

Synthetic

A substance produced by chemical synthesis, especially not of natural origin.

Tannin

A substance that acts as an astringent that helps seal tissues.

Terpene

One of a class of hydrocarbons with an empiric formula of $C10H16$, occurring in essential oils and resins.

Terpene less
An essential oil from which monoterpene hydrocarbons have been removed.

Tincture
An alcoholic solution prepared from herbal or perfume material.

Unguent
A soothing or healing salve, balm or ointment.

Vasoconstrictor
A substance that causes the vasoconstriction of blood vessels, which typically results in an increase in blood pressure and pupil dilation; vasodilatation is the opposite in which it relaxes the smooth muscle walls and causes the opening of blood vessels, lowering blood pressure.

Vein Tonic
A substance that improves and strengthens the functioning of blood vessels.

Vermifuge
An anathematic that expels parasitic worms from the body, by either stunning or killing them.

Viscosity
The degree of which a fluid moves and flows under an applied force. With carrier oils, it may be noted as "thin," or "thick," etc.

Volatile
A substance that is unstable and evaporates easily, such an essential oil.

Vulnerary
A remedy used for healing or treating wounds and helps to prevent tissue degeneration.

Warming
A substance that raises the temperature slightly.

Wound Healing
An agent that can assist in healing an injury, especially one in which the skin or another external surface that has been torn, pierced, cut, or otherwise broken.

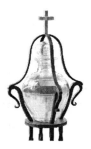

Bibliography

Totilo, Rebecca Park. *Therapeutic Blending With Essential Oil: Decoding the Healing Matrix of Aromatherapy.* Saint Petersburg: Rebecca at the Well Foundation, 2013. Print.

Totilo, Rebecca Park. *Anoint With Oil.* Saint Petersburg: Rebecca at the Well Foundation, 2014. Print.

Totilo, Rebecca Park. *Hebrew Wedding Customs.* Saint Petersburg: Rebecca at the Well Foundation, 2005.

Lost Tribes of Israel. WHBH. Public Broadcasting Service: Nova. Online. http://www.pbs.org/whbh/nova/israelifamilycohanium.html

Essential Oil Desk Reference (5th ed.). (2003). Lehi, UT: Life Science Publishing.

Null, Gary, PhD, Carolyn Dean MD, ND; Martin Feldman, MD, Debora Rasio, MD and Dorothy Smith, PhD. *"Death by Medicine."* WebDC.com. Nutrition Institute of America. Online. http://www.webdc.com/pdfs/deathbymedicine.pdf

Nesbit, Edward Planta. *Jesus An Essene.* (1895). Online. http://sacred-texts.com, http://bopsecrets.org

Stead, Miriam. *Egyptian Life.* Cambridge: Harvard University Press, 1609. Print.

Aykroyd, Dan. NBC. *Saturday Night Live.* New York: 1977. Television.

Schnaubelt, Kurt, PhD. *The Healing Intelligence of Essential Oils: The Science of Advanced Aromatherapy.* Rochester: Healing Arts Press, 2011. Print.

Cech, Misty Rae, ND. *"Essential Oils for a Strong Immune System."* PureInsideOut.com. Online. http://www.pureinsideout.com/essential-oils-for-cold-care-and-immune-system.html

Biblehub. (2015). Almond. Retrieved 08 26, 2015, from Biblehub.com: http://biblehub.com/topical/a/almond.htm

OrganicFacts.net. (2015). *Health Benefits of Bitter Almond oil.* Retrieved 08 26, 2015, from Organic Facts: https://www.organicfacts.net/health-benefits/essential-oils/health-benefits-of-bitter-almond-essential-oil.html

Parsons, J. (Unlisted). *Sign of The Almond Tree*. Retrieved 08 26, 2015, from Hebrew for Christians: http://www.hebrew4christians.com/Holidays/Winter_Holidays/Tu_B_shevat/Almond_Tree/almond_tree.html

Basil, S. (Unlisted). *In Creation of Terrestrial Animals*. Retrieved 08 26, 2015, from Buble Hub: http://biblehub.com/library/basil/basil_letters_and_select_works/homily_ix_the_creation_of.htm

Bible Hub. (n.d.). *Isaiah 28:25*. Retrieved 08 26, 2015, from Bible Hub: http://biblehub.com/isaiah/28-27.htm

BibleHub. (2015). *Hyssop*. Retrieved 08 26, 2015, from BibleHub: http://biblehub.com/topical/h/hyssop.htm

Botanical. (2015). *Fennel*. Retrieved 08 26, 2015, from Botanical: http://www.botanical.com/botanical/mgmh/f/fennel01.html

OrganicFacts.net. (2015). *Health Benefits of Marjoram Oil*. Retrieved 08 26, 2015, from Organic Facts: https://www.organicfacts.net/health-benefits/essential-oils/health-benefits-of-marjoram-essential-oil.html

Rivlin, R. S. (2001, 03). *Historical perspective on the use of garlic*. Retrieved 08 26, 2015, from Pubmed: http://www.ncbi.nlm.nih.gov/pubmed/11238795

Lawless, Julie. *The Encyclopedia of Essential Oils*. NewburyPort: Conari Press, 2013. Print.

OrganicFacts.net. *Health Benefits of Calamus Essential Oil*. Organicfacts.net. Online. https://www.organicfacts.

net/health-benefits/essential-oils/health-benefits-of-calamus-essential-oil.html

Eby, Preston J. Kingdom Bible Studies entitled, *The Ashes of a Red Heifer.* El Paso: Kingdom Bible Studies, 2012. Online http://www.kingdombiblestudies.org/ashes/ashes1.htm

Ratsch, Christian. *The Encyclopedia of Psychoactive Plants.* New York: Park Street Press, 1980. Print.

Habeeb.com. *Cedars of Lebanon, Cedars of the Lord.* Beirut: Habeeb.com, 2003-07. Online. http://www.habeeb.com/cedar.of.lebanon/cedar.of.lebanon.info.html

Kelly, Debra. 10 Truly Crazy Birds from World Mythology. Listverse.com. Online. http://listverse.com/2014/02/22/10-unusual-birds-from-world-mythology

Cooksley, Valerie, R.N. Aromatherapy: Soothing Remedies to Restore, Rejuvenate and Heal. Upper Saddle River: Prentice Hall, 2002. Print.

Ravindran, P.N., Nirmal Babu, K. and Shylaja M. *Cinnamon and Cassia*, Boca Raton: CRC Press, 2003. Paper.

Journal of Agricultural and Food Chemistry. ACS Publications, 2010. Online. http://pubs.acs.org/journal/jafcau

Gritman Essential Oils. (2015). *Garlic Essential Oil.* Retrieved 08 26, 2015, from Gritman.com: http://www.gritman.com/garlic-essential-oil.html

Herb Wisdom. (2015). *Marjoram (Origanum Majorana).* Retrieved 08 26, 2015, from Herb Wisdom: http://www.herbwisdom.com/herb-marjoram.html

Horn, S. (Unlisted). *Marjoram.* Retrieved 08 26, 2015, from Alington Agricultural Gardening Club: http://www.aogc.org/plants/herbs/marjoram.htm

Jewish Virtual Library. (Unlisted). *Spices.* Retrieved 08 26, 2015, from Jewish Virtual Library: http://www.jewishvirtuallibrary.org/jsource/judaica/ejud_0002_0019_0_18967.html

Oil Health Benefits. (2015). *Almond Oil.* Retrieved 08 26, 2015, from Oil Health Benefits : http://oilhealthbenefits.com/almond-oil/

Chillemi, Stacey. *The Complete Herbal Guide: A Natural Approach to Healing the Body.* Raleigh: Lulu, 2011. Paper.

Arieh Moussaieff, Neta Rimmerman, Tatiana Bregman, Alex Straiker, Christian C. Felder, Shai Shoham, Yoel Kashman, Susan M. Huang, Hyosang Lee, Esther Shohami, Ken Mackie, Michael J. Caterina, J. Michael Walker, Ester Fride and Raphael Mechoulam. *Incensole acetate, an incense component, elicits psychoactivity by activating TRPV3 channels in the brain.* FASEB Journal,

2008. Online. http://www.fasebj.org/content/22/8/3024.
long

Roberts, John. *Animal Health at the Crossroads - Preventing, Detecting and Diagnosing Animal Diseases.* Virginia-Maryland College of Veterinary Medicine, 2006. Online. http://www.vetmed.vt.edu/news/vs/jan06/

Complementary and Alternative Medicine. University of Oklahoma, 2009. Online. http://bmccomplementalternmed.biomedcentral.com/articles/10.1186/1472-6882-9-6

Raychaudhuri, Sibi. *Frankincense AKBA Potent Anti-Inflammatory Properties.* University of California. Online. http://undergroundhealthreporter.com/herbal-arthritis-remedies-frankincense-can-help-diminish-pain-from-arthritis/#axzz42vywd7zN

Stewart, David, Ph.D., D.N.M. *The Chemistry of Essential Oils Made Simple: God's love manifest in molecules.* Grand Rapids: CARE Publications, 2005. Paper.

Stewart, David, PhD., D.N.M. Healing Oils of the Bible. Grand Rapids: Care Publications, 2003. Paper.

Stewart, Vabener, Dr. Seminar Course. University of Izmir. Turkey, 1996.

David, Metzudat. The commentary by Metzudat David ("The Bulwark of David") Zolkiev, 1862. Online. http://schoolebooklibrary.com/article/whebn0005524018/david%20ben%20solomon%20ibn%20abi%20zimra

Frazer, James. *The Golden Bough*. United Kingdom: Macmillan Press, 1890. Paper.

Hepper, F. Nigel, *The Encyclopedia of Bible Plants*, 1992. Paper.

Rafi, Mohamed, Dr. *Myrrh Anti-cancer and Effective for Prevention and Treatment of Breast and Prostrate Cancer.* Journal of Natural Products. Rutgers University, 2009.

Analgesic Effects of Myrrh, Nature Magazine. 1996.

Murr, Andrew. *A Winning Equation.* Newsweek Magazine, 2006. Online. http://www.newsweek.com/winning-equation-108969

Higley, A. & Conni, *Reference Guide to Essential Oils.* Abundant Health, 2014. Paper.

Ledoux, Dr. Joseph. New York Medical University.

Cromie, William. *Researchers Sniff out Secrets in Smell.* Harvard University Gazette.

Forbes, A. *Tacuinum Sanitatis'. Health and Well Being: A Medieval Guide.* Raleigh: Lulu, 2013. Paper.

The Life of Jesus Christ Collectors Edition, Disc 1. Courtesy of Diamond Entertainment, copyrighted. Video.

Dietrich Gumbel, Ph.D.

Oliver, C. R. Dr. *Solomon's Secret.* The Woodlands: Zadok Publications, 2006. Paper.

Aura Cacia, http://auracacia.com. Online.

Chernobyl Fall Out: Apocalyptic Tale. New York Times. New York, 1986. Online.

Bouw, Gerald D. *Essay on Wormwood.* Online.

Adams, J. *Hideous Absinthe: A History of the Devil in a bottle.* Madison: University of Wisconsin Press, 2004. Paper.

Books by
REBECCA PARK TOTILO

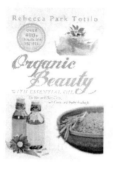

ORGANIC BEAUTY WITH ESSENTIAL OIL: OVER 400+ HOMEMADE RECIPES FOR NATURAL SKIN CARE, HAIR CARE , BATH & BODY PRODUCTS

Sweep aside all those harmful chemically-based cosmetics and make your own organic bath and body products at home with the magic of potent essential oils! In this book, you'll find a luxurious array of over 400 Eco-friendly recipes that call for breathtaking fragrances and soothing, rich organic ingredients satisfying you head to toe. Included you'll find helpful hints so you can have the confidence knowing which essential oil to use and how much when creating your own body scrub, lip butter, or lotion bar! Discover how easy it is to make bath treats like fragrant shower gels, dreamy bubble baths, luscious creams and lotions, deep cleansing masks and facials for literally pennies using only a few essential oils and ingredients from your own kitchen with Organic Beauty with Essential Oil.

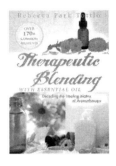

THERAPEUTIC BLENDING WITH ESSENTIAL OIL: DECODING THE HEALING MATRIX OF AROMATHERAPY

Now you can safely create natural therapeutic blends that will impact your mood and health and best of all, promote well-being. Therapeutic Blending With Essential Oil unlocks the healing power of essential oils and guides you through the intricate matrix of aromatherapy, with a compilation of over 170 common ailments. Discover how to properly formulate a blend for any physical or emotional symptom with easy to follow customizable recipes. Now, you can make your own personalized massage oils, hand and body lotions, bath gels, compresses, salve ointments, smelling salts, nasal inhalers and more. This exhaustive guide takes all the guesswork out of blending essential oils from how many drops to include in a blend, to working with and measuring thick oils, to how often to apply it for acute or chronic conditions.

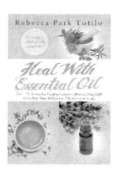

HEAL WITH ESSENTIAL OIL: NATURE'S MEDICINE CABINET

Using essential oils drawn from nature's own medicine cabinet of flowers, trees, seeds and roots, man can tap into God's healing power to heal oneself from almost any pain. Find relief from many conditions and rejuvenate the body. With over 125 recipes, this practical guide will walk you through in the most easy-to-understand form how to treat common ailments with your essential oils for everyday living. Filled with practical advice on therapeutic blending of oils and safety, a directory of the most effective oils for common ailments and easy to follow remedies chart, and prescriptive blends for aches, pains and sicknesses.

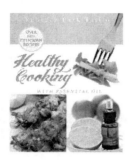

HEALTHY COOKING WITH ESSENTIAL OIL

Imagine transforming an everyday dish into something extraordinary – using only a drop or two of essential oil can enliven everything from soups, salads, to main dishes and desserts. Boasting flavor and fragrance, these intense essences can turn a dull, boring meal into something appetizing and delicious. Essential oils are fun, easy-to-use and beneficial, compared to the traditional stale, dried herbs and spices found in most pantries today. Healthy food should never be thought of as mere fuel for the body, it should be enjoyed as a multi-sensory experience that brings therapeutic value as well as nourishment. For years we have limited the use of essential oils to scented candles and soaps, in the belief that they were unsafe to consume (and some are!). However, more people are realizing the value of using pure essential oils to enhance their diet. In Healthy Cooking With Essential Oil, you will learn how cooking with essential oils can open up a wealth of creative opportunities in the kitchen. Packed with over 100+ traditional recipes to experiment with, this cookbook also includes an exhaustive directory of essential oils and herbs commonly used in cooking and some of their therapeutic properties, blending techniques for creating favorite essential oil flavor groups, quick pinch substitution guides for spices and herbs, ways to use hydrosols for marinades, dressings, and dipping oils, easy, superfast recipes for making your own seasoned and flavored salts, and charts galore for knowing which essential oils to use for smoothies, flavored honeys, and more!

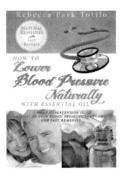

HOW TO LOWER BLOOD PRESSURE NATURALLY WITH ESSENTIAL OIL

One out of three adults have it, and another one-third don't realize it. Oftentimes, it goes undetected for years. Even those who take multiple medications for it still don't have it under control. It's no secret – high blood pressure is rampant in America. High blood pressure, or hypertension, has become a household term. Between balancing meds and monitoring diets though, are the true causes – and best treatments – hidden in the shadows? In How to Lower Blood Pressure Naturally With Essential Oil, Rebecca Park Totilo sheds light on what high blood pressure is, the causes and symptoms of high blood pressure, and which essential oils regulate blood pressure and how to use essential oils as a natural, alternative method. Included within the pages of this book are simple blending techniques, dilution charts, and a wide variety of recipes for everyday use such as the Heart Plus Roll-On Blend and the Love My Heart Massage Oil. Get creative with the basic blend recipes and discover your new favorite "medication." With no side effects and no prescription necessary, essential oils offer a healthy aromatic and therapeutic option for controlling your blood pressure.

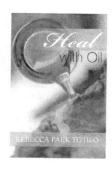

HEAL WITH OIL: HOW TO USE THE ESSENTIAL OILS OF ANCIENT SCRIPTURE

Buried within the passages of scriptures lies a hidden treasure – possibly every man's answer to illness and disease. Now you can learn their secret and discover how to transform your life and walk in divine health. In this exhaustive study by Certified Aromatherapist Rebecca Park Totilo you will discover each oil's rich biblical history and/or pagan roots, their spiritual significance, symbolism and hidden meanings behind each bible oil, and their healing properties including traditional uses, medicinal properties, and applications. You will find numerous scripture references with Hebrew or Greek meanings, along with their usage based on science and research, with over 30 essential oil datasheets showing the breakdown of the chemical components, helping you to identify the oil's therapeutic benefits with safety information.

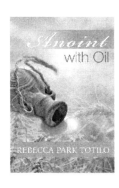

ANOINT WITH OIL

Throughout the Middle Ages, the church persecuted anyone who made ointments, oils, or unguents -- calling them "magic potions." Considered a capital offense, apothecaries mislabeled as witches were penalized for this crime by being burnt at the stake. This tragedy should not have been, as for thousands of years before, oils and incense were not only important but also necessary in healing, worship, and even daily hygiene. In Anoint With Oil, Rebecca Park Totilo shares an aromatic and therapeutic journey through the scriptures, showing the purpose of anointing with oil, the methods used in the Bible and their symbolism, the ingredients of the holy anointing oil, and the uses of essential oils mentioned in the Old and New Testaments. Discover new scents within these pages and find out why the right ear, right thumb, and right big toe were anointed, what the mysterious fifth ingredient of the holy anointing oil was, which oils did Jesus anoint with, and who is qualified to perform the anointing ritual.

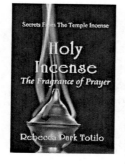

QETORET (HOLY INCENSE): THE FRAGRANCE OF PRAYER

The burning of the Qetoret (Holy Incense) was central to all of the ceremonies conducted in the Temple as key component required under the Law of Moses. As a close-guarded secret passed down from generation to generation, this particular formula for Holy Incense was made only for the worship of the Lord and required certain rituals in preparation. In this exhaustive study, Rebecca identifies the spices used and the exact amounts and manner in which they were prepared and presented in ceremony. In Qetoret: The Fragrance of Prayer, you will learn the importance of "burning your Holy Incense before God" and the necessary ingredients for effectual prayer. Discover what each ingredient of the Qetoret (Holy Incense) symbolizes and how your prayer can be a sweet savour to our Heavenly Father and bring change to your current situation or circumstance.

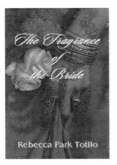

THE FRAGRANCE OF THE BRIDE

The Fragrance of the Bride awakens your senses to the spiritual significance of the fragrances mentioned in the Song of Solomon and how these aromatic spices draw believers into a deeper understanding of their Messiah. Each chief spice emits the "sweet aroma" and characteristics the Bride of Christ must possess in order to be made ready as His wife.

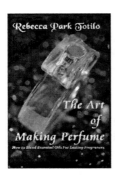

THE ART OF MAKING PERFUME

With a ton of recipes and helpful hints on perfume making, you'll discover how to make homemade perfumes, body sprays, aftershave colognes, floral waters and much more using pure essential oils. Rebecca shares insider secrets from the beauty industry how to develop your very own signature fragrance. Topics include: History of Perfumery, The Ancient Art of Extracting Oils & Making Perfumes, Easy-to-Follow Steps on Perfume Making, Perfumes for Holistic Healing & Well-Being, Perfumes Kids Can Make, Perfume For Your Dog, & How to Start Your Own Perfume Business.

CPSIA information can be obtained at www.ICGtesting.com
Printed in the USA
LVOW08s0214100616

491967LV00017B/51/P